THE THERAPEUTIC POWER OF THE MAGGIE'S CENTRE

This book is about the therapeutic environment of the Maggie's centre and it explores the many ways the centre accomplishes its goal. With unconventional architecture as required by the design brief, combined with Maggie's psychological support programme, this special health facility fosters extraordinary therapeutic effects in people, to such a degree that one can truly speak of the therapeutic power of what goes on in these centres.

After going back over the story of the Maggie's centre, the book reveals its basic tenets: Maggie's *Therapeutikos* (the-mind-as-important-as-the-body), the Architectural Brief, and the 'Client-Architect-Users' Triad. It continues by laying bare Maggie's synergy—between people and place—increasing the users' psychological flexibility and helping them to tolerate what was intolerable before. Although comfort and atmosphere are paramount, they are not enough to define the therapeutic environment of the Maggie's centre. It is only by looking at neuroscience, which can provide us with scientific explanations for empathy, feelings, and emotions, and only by considering space as being neither neutral nor empty but filled with forces that envelop people in an 'embodied experience', that we can explain what generates *wellbeing* in a Maggie's centre.

The conclusion of the book critically evaluates the Maggie's centre as a model to be applied to other healthcare facilities and to architecture in general. It is essential reading for any student or professional involved in therapeutic environments.

Caterina Frisone was awarded a PhD and was Associate Lecturer in Interior Architecture at Oxford Brookes University, UK. She is currently the Scientific Director of the Postgraduate programme 'Master in Architecture and Health' at the Università Iuav di Venezia, Italy.

"The role of emotions and feelings for a person left alone in that limbo that follows a cancer diagnosis is why Maggie Keswick Jencks started her pilot project for a centre with a human element at its core which, since 1996, has continued to grow to help more and more people with cancer. Explaining our philosophy with strength and passion, this book promotes Maggie's values that hopefully go beyond health-care and reach a wider architectural audience."

Dame Laura Lee, *Maggie's CEO*

"And I came in and I was in the centre for about three hours, and the initial feeling of walking through that door, and just looking up and seeing it, was there even then and felt that powerful, that I was in a powerful place. I think I felt I was in a safe place. And that's what I feel when I've come into Maggie's, I feel safe, here."

Malita, *Maggie's Dundee visitor*

"I couldn't believe my cancer diagnosis, but then I thought 'I can come here every day! I can sit in a corner and cry some time, yeah!' I swear to God, if I didn't have it, I don't think I would be ok as I am."

Elizabeth, *Maggie's Barts visitor*

"This is not the business of healthcare, but it is the business of the spirit. And it really is a very spiritual place, in a non-religious way."

Carol, *Maggie's Oldham visitor*

THE THERAPEUTIC POWER OF THE MAGGIE'S CENTRE

Experience, Design and Wellbeing, Where Architecture Meets Neuroscience

Caterina Frisone

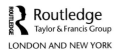
Routledge
Taylor & Francis Group

LONDON AND NEW YORK

Designed cover image: Maggie's Edinburgh (1996). Architect: Richard Murphy. Photograph credit: Alan Forbes.

First published 2024
by Routledge
4 Park Square, Milton Park, Abingdon, Oxon OX14 4RN

and by Routledge
605 Third Avenue, New York, NY 10158

Routledge is an imprint of the Taylor & Francis Group, an informa business

British Library Cataloguing-in-Publication Data
A catalogue record for this book is available from the British Library

Library of Congress Cataloging-in-Publication Data
A catalog record has been requested for this book

ISBN: 9781032154572 (hbk)
ISBN: 9781032155265 (pbk)
ISBN: 9781003244516 (ebk)

DOI: 10.4324/9781003244516

Typeset in Times New Roman
by codeMantra

*To my parents, Annamaria and Placido Frisone,
who taught me to be curious, courageous and tireless in
the search for wellbeing.*

CONTENTS

PREFACE

This preface aims to explain the background of the book and highlight its main purpose, which is to raise awareness in the reader of what a therapeutic environment is (not necessarily in the health sector) in order to be able to recognise it in any architecture that makes one feel well. Analysing the therapeutic environment of the Maggie's centre, in addition to telling what generates and defines it, the book critically evaluates Maggie's as a model to be applied to other health and non-health facilities, and, possibly, to architecture in general.

The book stems from my doctoral thesis "The Role of Architecture in the Therapeutic Environment: The Case of the Maggie's Cancer Care Centre" in which I investigated from an architectural point of view the postulate of Maggie's Psychologist Lead Lesley Howells (2016), who argues that "the synergy between people and place enables psychological flexibility", i.e. the psychological impact generated by the bespoke architecture of the Maggie's centre, in synergy with the psychological support offered by Maggie's staff, allows a flexible state of mind in its users to constitute a therapeutic environment. In other words, I assessed the beneficial effect on people with cancer and their carers of what they call 'healing architecture', in the case study of the Maggie's centre.

Although in the world there are numerous examples of innovative healthcare facilities that have achieved good results, the architecture of the Maggie's centre is one of a kind and within the British National Health Service (NHS) this awareness is growing fast, along with the curiosity about its success. Seen from the perspective of the person with cancer, the main reason for this success is the sense of safety.

The word safe is what comes to mind to describe the Maggie's centre. You are safe to talk about cancer or not. When you're in the world, and you have cancer, you can't talk to your friends and family because they're stressed out for you.

And besides, nobody understands if they're not going through it. But, when you come here, everybody is in the same boat, everybody just talks openly about it, and there is a sense of relief.

(Move-along_no.6 Barts)

In addition to feeling safe, according to Maggie's organisation, as soon as they enter, 'visitors' (this is how people with cancer, family and friends are called alike) feel a sense of calm and control, which are the expression of the therapeutic effects released from the environment. At the same time, together with it, other types of emotions begin to emerge that lead them to say, often in tears: "I don't know what it is", "I can't explain it". Since these emotional phenomena observed by the staff had never been investigated and many therapeutic effects had not yet been interpreted, with the mission to verify them and, in general, to understand what exactly generates wellbeing in a Maggie's centre, in 2018 I started my doctoral research.

To this end, I first visited all the Maggie's centres and interviewed 12 Maggie's architects about their interpretation of the Architectural Brief, the programme the architects receive when asked to design their centre. Second, I immersed myself for almost four months in three of the 23—today 30—existing centres to investigate how visitors live in everyday life, adopting phenomenology as a method of knowledge. Once I had completed my ethnographic work and tested the effectiveness of 'the synergy between people and place' from an architectural point of view, I was able to confirm that the Maggie's centre is a therapeutic environment, that is, the meeting point between architecture and people (*Howells, 16.06.2017*). Despite this confirmation, however, I felt that it wasn't just this that generated wellbeing in Maggie's visitors and that I had to investigate further.

Similar to Lesley Howells' analysis, previous studies on the 'healing architecture' of the Maggie's centre had attributed the therapeutic nature of the building to the synergistic action of "generators of architectural atmospheres", i.e. the combination of materials, light, colour and shape of the buildings (Martin, Nettleton and Buse, 2019), together with the good care of the staff. However, no one had gone further in explaining *why* this synergy was generated, *where* it came from and, therefore, *what* was the true source of the therapeutic effects of the Maggie's centre. Through the in-depth study of the Architectural Brief and the adoption of phenomenology—which I initially intended to use only as a method of investigation in my ethnographic work, but which I later discovered to be relevant to various aspects of Maggie's therapeutic environment—my research took a turn. And, in this, distance has helped.

Once I left the three centres and transcribed the conversations with people, thinking back to my daily experiences there, one day—while cooking!—I succeeded to find the answer I was looking for. I understood that the secrets were hidden in the movement that the space of the Maggie's centre generates and, therefore, in the Architectural Brief from which the dynamic space derives. Since, in addition to providing an understanding of experience, phenomenology also explains how the environment influences our visual perception and behaviour, as suggested by Sternberg (2009), along the way, I decided to explore neuroscience. Within my PhD theoretical framework, the importance of adding this discipline to those of psychology, geography and sociology has helped improve my understanding of how people's brains perceive and respond to the built environment.

Wanting to deepen my understanding of the impact that the therapeutic environment has on Maggie's users and how they respond to it biologically, in writing this book I turned to neuroscience primarily for two aspects: that of 'perception', i.e. the experience triggered by movement and in which the brain serves to "predict the future, to anticipate the consequences of action" (Berthoz, 2000, p. 1) (scientifically demonstrated by the discovery of mirror neurons) and that of 'emotions and feelings' in the experiential process of which, again thanks to movement, the related brain structures are "those necessary for reasoning and to culminate in decision making" (Damasio, 1994, p. 39). Both of these aspects go back to the origins of the existence of humans and animals—beings dependent on their natural environment or *Umwelt* (=surrounding world)—out of the need for survival and reproduction, improving over time the brain's ability to investigate the world, planning and deciding, for example, whether to 'fight' or 'fly'. By bringing to the reader's attention people's behaviours from a biological point of view in response to Maggie's dynamic space and unconventional architecture, this book aims to explain the ability of the Maggie's centre to generate emotional phenomena and, therefore, why we can talk about its therapeutic power.

Although there is already an increasing number of publications in 'Architecture and Neuroscience', paradoxically, in the healthcare sector, there is not enough literature on today's case studies that correlates the spatial and material characteristics that a healthcare environment must have and the positive effects on users and on their immune system (Sternberg, 2009). This book on the study of a current and easily accessible healthcare facility, such as that of the Maggie's centre, has the advantage of facilitating the reader, professional or student of architecture, layman or not of neuroscience, in understanding the relationship between the two disciplines, highlighting the advantages that this blend would bring, encouraging greater consideration in future projects. Aware of having just begun to delve into neuroscience, in this book I wanted to open a door to the vast knowledge in this field, leaving the reader free to go further in individual research. However, since other perspectives that look at neuroscience applied to architecture and healthcare are also needed, this book is actually an even broader invitation to delve into the topic.

Reflecting my passion for architecture and interest in the human experiences it generates, this book also has the ultimate goal of extending the essence of Maggie's model to other healthcare and non-healthcare facilities and, beyond the research of the Maggie's centre, to architecture in general. Besides hoping to be a good reading for doctors, psychologists and neuroscientists, urging them to think more about human needs in the architectural space of healthcare, in fact, this book aims to stimulate a new way of perceiving architecture. If it reaches the interest of ordinary people, who as users learn how to recognise an architecture that makes one feel good or bad, becoming more critical and demanding, in the long run, they will contribute to triggering that mechanism by which architects and builders will be pushed to design and build a better built environment.

As a final note to the reader, I would like to explain that although it started as "Maggie's Cancer Caring Centre" (Jencks, 2015), over time the charity has abandoned 'Cancer Caring' and then 'Centre', becoming first the Maggie's Centre and only recently Maggie's. However, in this book, essentially architectural, to highlight the physicality of the place, I will keep using 'centre' for the building but with the lowercase 'c' to help the organisation to define themselves only as 'Maggie's'.

ACKNOWLEDGEMENTS

The five years I spent doing research on the Maggie's centre have profoundly marked my life. First of all, as a person. Meeting Charles Jencks, discussing many topics with him, but above all hearing directly from him many stories on his wife Maggie, was a source of enrichment that forged my mind indelibly. Moreover, meeting women like Dame Laura Lee (Maggie's CEO), Marcia Blakenham (Maggie's best friend and Maggie's co-client with Laura Lee) and Lesley Howells (Maggie's Psychologist Lead)—all three characterised by a beautiful smile behind which lies strength, courage, strategy, intelligence, far-sightedness, determination, commitment and love for others—gave me a new perspective. Therefore, a special memory goes to Charles (who left us too soon, in 2019), while a warm thanks goes to Laura, Marcia and Lesley, along with the one addressed to the Maggie's Advisory Board (now remodelled into the Professional Advisors Group), of which Lesley Howells is a member. Thanks to Laura Lee, I was also able to meet and interview 12 Maggie's architects, who enriched my research not only with their knowledge and experience but also with their generosity by opening to me the doors of their archives. For dedicating their time and attention to my research, I deeply thank Richard Murphy (RMA); David Page (Page\Park); Frank Gehry (Gehry Partners); Ivan Harbour (RSHP); Ellen van Loon (OMA); Piers Gough (CZWG); Bjørg Aabø (Snøhetta); Darron Haylock (Foster+Parners); Wendy James and Jo Spittles (Gabers&James); Alex de Rijke and Jasmin Sohi (dRMM); Steven Holl and Chris McVoy (SHA); Benedetta Tagliabue and Joan Callís (EMBT). I also thank Darren Hawkes, the landscape architect of Maggie's Forth Valley and Maggie's Barts whom I met during my ethnographic work and who provided me with his perspectives on therapeutic gardens. If the architectural content of this book is therefore based on conversations with these architects, I would like to let the other Maggie's architects know that, although they have perhaps not been cited enough here, they have, through their buildings (which I have carefully visited), equally contributed to and influenced the outcome of this book.

I also want to thank all the people who work for Maggie's organisation, especially the management staff and their collaborators who generously gave me their time to organise visits to the centres, interviews with the architects and collect materials. Of course, another huge thanks must go to the operational staff of the single centres. Here I have to open a big parenthesis. To say 'special' is still not enough. As one of my participants once said, the people who work at Maggie's are just those 'of a certain type'. I start with the staff who have been active during my ethnographic fieldwork (September–December 2019) at Maggie's Dundee, thanking Lesley, Karen, Hannah, Sian, Joy, Nancy, Sheila, Laura, Victoria, Moira, Jeanne and Peter. I follow with the Maggie's Oldham team, thanking Trish, Laura-Jayne, Suzanne, Geraldine, Laura, Tom, Diana, Carol, Lynna, Norma, Val, John, Stef, Jackie and Jean. I conclude by the Maggie's Barts team, thanking Michael, Monique, Janet, Mary, Leah, Carrie, Jamie, Hannah, Steven, Julia, Carolyne, Beatrice, Patricia, Deborah and Diana. To this list, I add all the staff of the centres I visited during the photo shoots for this book. Indeed, I also want to thank my photographer Marco, who was able to capture the therapeutic power of Maggie's centre with images that amaze me every time I look at them: almost three dimensional, they penetrate the brain deeply, doing something to our minds that other photos don't. But nothing would ever have been possible without Maggie's visitors—people with cancer, their families and friends—who are the most important people in this book. So, last but not least, I want to thank everyone who responded to my cooperation request and actively participated in my survey, accepting my presence with flexibility and openness despite their illness. My infinite thanks go to them together with a message of affection, letting them know that they made my experience special and that they will remain an indelible memory in my heart.

As a development of my PhD thesis—albeit ultimately something very different—of course, this book owes much to my experience as a researcher undertaken at Oxford Brookes University, which was both rich and pioneering. Indeed, in 2017, when I planned this adventure, the high-level academic research Brookes required was uncharted territory for me. In line with the orientation of the OBU School of Architecture, my PhD thesis on the relationship between the design of the built environment and people's wellbeing—i.e. my research on the Maggie's centre—has gone beyond the mere idea of considering the environment as a place capable of enhancing the human experience. And this was possible thanks to the work carried out by a truly exceptional supervisory team, made up of Cathrine Brun, Andrea Placidi and Lesley Howells (Maggie's Psychologist Lead): they all pushed me to go beyond myself. A special thanks goes to Andrea who continued to help me even by reading the entire draft of this book, however not failing to put me to hard test. In the academy the challenge is always at a high level and, in this, the confrontation with Alain Berthoz and Laura Boella and the approval by Susan

Brennan—all honourable academics who corrected some neuroscience sections in this book—was a demanding challenge but also a great honour to have it.

Without forgetting the more deeply human side of this experience and what inspired it, I conclude by thanking my supportive family, including my four wonderful daughters who have encouraged me to continue and whom I hope to inspire at least for my stubbornness. I also remember my wonderful mother, over a hundred years old yet lucid, knowledgeable and wise, who helped me correct, simplify and clarify the concepts of my doctorate and who, together with my father, supported and encouraged me throughout my life. My last thoughts go to my brother Francesco, who died of brain cancer in 2013 at the age of 55. There are no Maggie's centres in Italy. Had they been there during his illness, he would have lived his last year of life in a more dignified way. This is why my future commitment is to create a Maggie's centre in Italy.

TERMS USED IN
THE MAGGIE'S CENTRE

Maggie's centre: the building

Maggie's: the organisation

Maggie Keswick: founder (1941–1995†)

Charles Jencks: Maggie Keswick's husband and Maggie's co-founder (1939–2019†)

Dame Laura Lee: Maggie Keswick's oncological nurse (1993–95), Maggie's CEO and Co-Client (1996 ongoing)

Marcia Blakenham: Maggie Keswick's best friend and Maggie's Co-Client

Maggie's Legacy: President, Vice Presidents, Centre Board Chairs, Honorary Patrons, Ambassadors, Board of Directors, Executive Board, Architecture Co-Clients, Centre Staff

Architecture Co-Clients: Laura Lee and Marcia Blakenham

Blueprint for a Cancer Caring Centre: text by Maggie Keswick (1995) on which the Architectural Brief is based

A View from the Front Line: Maggie's description of what it is like to be diagnosed with cancer and then cope with it (1995), updated by Marcia Blakenham (2007)

Architectural Brief (1998, 2003, 2007): Maggie Keswick's philosophy and instructions for the architects

Architectural and Landscape Brief (2015): the updated version of the Architectural Brief (2007)

Maggie's Architects: all the architects who designed or are designing a Maggie's centre

Maggie's Programme of Support (*Practical, Lifestyle, Emotional*): the support programme offered by Maggie's organisation

Users: Visitors and Staff

Visitors: people with cancer, their family and friends

Centre Staff: Maggie's (Centre Head, Clinical Psychologist, Cancer Support Specialist, Benefits Advisor, Fundraiser), External (Relaxation Therapist, Sessional Staff, Volunteers)

Centre Head, Psychologist and Cancer Support Specialist: three basic clinical staff figures

Benefits Advisor, Fundraiser: two basic non-clinical staff figures

Centre Head: oversees everything that happens in the centre, supporting the needs of people with cancer, managing the support programme and mentoring the staff

Clinical Psychologist: supports people to address complex psychological issues through a range of therapeutic approaches

Cancer Support Specialist (CSS): welcomes newcomers and offers high-quality individual and group support to centre visitors

Volunteers in a centre: people who provide a warm welcome and cup of tea to visitors or help with fundraising

Maggie's Kitchen Table Day: a fundraising initiative where people are asked to arrange a meeting around a table for dinner or tea

Maggie's to Maggie's: run or walk between centres to raise funds

NOTE ON THE TEXT

All references enclosed in brackets and written regularly (e.g., Jencks, 2015) can be found in the 'References' at the end of each chapter. All interviews, conferences, symposiums, which are not public, are enclosed in brackets and written in italics (e.g., *Aabø, 02.11.2018* or *Move-along_no.1 Dundee*) and are limited to the details enclosed in brackets. The asterisk* next to a reference in brackets means that I translated the sentence from Italian (e.g., Gallese, 2009, p. 9*). Further supporting material can be found in the Appendices (e.g., Appendix I). Data on the Maggie's centre is available online at www.maggies.org.

Due to the nature of this research, participant names will remain anonymous except for those who have kindly endorsed this book. For more information about my PhD research see https://doi.org/10.24384/0ejy-7815.

1
INTRODUCTION

Premise

I remember just starting the interview with Maggie's co-clients, Laura Lee and Marcia Blakenham, and discovering to my surprise that, other than for its gardens, neither of them had ever used the terms 'healing' or 'therapeutic' to define the Maggie's centre.

> I think we never say to someone 'we want you to create a healing environment' at all, because that would be awful and assumptive that 'you need to be healed' and 'we are going to heal you in this environment'. I think that's sort of an arrogant concept.
>
> (*Lee, 18.05.2019*)

With my research entirely focused on the therapeutic environment of the Maggie's centre, at that moment, I felt a real shock. For the first time, in more than a year of work, I found myself faced with a major obstacle which naturally raised fundamental doubts, in addition to the dilemma, whether, due to the possible 'passive' or 'clinical' interpretation of the term, 'therapeutic' was not the right adjective for a Maggie's centre. Without anticipating too much about how I found my way after this episode, I can safely say that this 'breakdown' led me to unveil one of the big secrets behind the Maggie's centre.

At that time, I had already encountered cancer first-hand with my brother's illness and death in 2013 and had heard the story of Maggie Keswick and her centre directly from her husband, Charles Jencks. I had met him by chance at a conference at UCL in London in November 2015 and we immediately became friends. Glad to accept the invitation to his home in Holland Park, that is how I then got to learn

DOI: 10.4324/9781003244516-1

about the magical world he had shared with his wife Maggie until 1995. Designed by Charles with the help of his former students, the Cosmic House (1980s) is a concentrate of symbols and metaphors, an extreme example of how unconventional architecture manages to distract and intrigue with the aim of making people feel good. There is a nice video of the Cosmic House, now home to the Jencks Foundation and Museum, which is worth watching [Alice Dousova- Zuketa LTD (2023)].

Starting with the visits to all Maggie's centres, with the exception of the two in Hong Kong and Japan, by early November 2018 I had seen all 19 buildings in the UK and the one in Spain, to complete the tour with those that were subsequently opened, between 2020 and 2023 (Table 1.1). After these visits, I had the definitive confirmation of what I was gradually discovering, namely that at Maggie's, "the architecture is there for you". Alex de Rijke (dRMM), the first of the 12 Maggie's architects I interviewed, explained to me that people who enter a Maggie's centre get the very clear message that "design is a form of care". "It is really about letting architecture speak about care, and that is what design is" (*de Rijke, 17.12.2018*).

TABLE 1.1 List of the built and upcoming Maggie's centres (1996 onwards)

	Name of the Centre	*Country*	*Maggie's Architect*	*Year*
1	Maggie's Edinburgh	Scotland	Richard Murphy OBE (Richard Murphy Architects)	1996
2	Maggie's Glasgow, The Gatehouse Office	Scotland	David Page, Karen Nugent (Page\Park)	2002
3	Maggie's Dundee	Scotland	Frank Gehry (Gehry Partners)	2003
4	Maggie's Highlands	Scotland	David Page, Andy Bateman (Page\Park)	2005
5	Maggie's Fife	Scotland	Zaha Hadid (Zaha Hadid Architects)	2006
6	Maggie's West London	England	Ivan Harbour, Richard Rogers (RSHP)	2008
7	Maggie's Cheltenham	England	Sir Richard MacCormac (MJP Architects)	2010
8	Maggie's Glasgow Gartnavel	Scotland	Rem Koolhaas, Ellen van Loon (OMA)	2011
9	Maggie's Nottingham	England	Piers Gough (CZWG Architects) and Paul Smith Ltd (interior design)	2011
10	Maggie's Swansea	Wales	Kisho Kurokawa Architects and Garbers&James	2011
11	Maggie's Newcastle	England	Ted Cullinan (Cullinan Studio)	2013
12	Maggie's Aberdeen	Scotland	Bjørg Aabø (Snøhetta)	2013
13	Maggie's Hong Kong	HK	Frank Gehry (Gehry Partners)	2013
14	Maggie's Merseyside (demolished) substituted by Maggie's Wirral (2021)	England	Carmody Groarke and Dennis Swain (HB Architects)	2014

(*Continued*)

TABLE 1.1 (Continued)

	Name of the Centre	Country	Maggie's Architect	Year
15	Maggie's Lanarkshire	Scotland	Reiach and Hall Architects	2014
16	Maggie's Oxford	England	Chris Wilkinson (WilkinsonEyre)	2014
17	Maggie's Manchester	England	Foster+Partners	2016
18	Maggie's Tokyo	Japan	Cosmos More and Nikken Sekkei Ltd. coordinated by Tsutomu Abe	2016
19	Maggie's Forth Valley	Scotland	Wendy James, Thore Garbers (Garbers&James)	2017
20	Maggie's Oldham	England	Alex de Rijke, Jasmin Sohi (dRMM Architects)	2017
21	Maggie's Barts	England	Steven Holl (SHA)	2017
22	Kálida Barcelona	Spain	Benedetta Tagliabue, Joan Callis (EMBT)	2019
23	Maggie's Cardiff	Wales	Biba Dow, Alun Jones (Dow Jones Architects)	2019
24	Maggie's at The Royal Marsden	England	Ab Rogers (Ab Rogers Design)	2019
25	Maggie's Yorkshire	England	Thomas Heatherwick (Heatherwick Studio)	2019
26	Maggie's Southampton	England	Amanda Levete (AL_A)	2021
27	Maggie's The Royal Free	England	Daniel Libeskind (Studio Libeskind)	2024
28	Maggie's Northampton	England	Stephen Marshall (Stephen Marshall Architects)	TBC
29	Maggie's Coventry	England	Jamie Fobert (Jamie Fobert Architects)	TBC
30	Maggie's Cambridge	England	Níall McLaughlin (Níall McLaughlin Architects)	TBC

In this regard, the Maggie's centre represents a significant example. In synergy with the practical and psychological support offered by Maggie's organisation, the striking architecture of its built environment, which is a requirement of the programme and one of the reasons for its success, helps people with cancer to accept the disease, something that was intolerable before. This attitude stems from a state of psychological flexibility contained in Maggie Keswick Jencks' quote: "Above all, what matters is not to lose the joy of living for fear of dying" (1994). Receiving compassion and safety, but certainly not "a pat on the head" (Blakenham, 2007, p. 1), people with cancer find the strength to face reality and react and, without fighting a past that no longer exists or a future that could never happen, they come to accept their new condition.

To this end, the architects' experience is essential to create unconventional and uplifting architectures that stimulate curiosity and imagination, involving people in a continuous "spatial interaction rather than walls" (*Howells, 16.06.2017*). In a space that allows sociality and intimacy at the same time, openness, combined with active people inside, is essential to make people feel included, becoming a catalyst for the psychological healing process. As the organisation states, it is based on evidence that the architecture combined with the support programme founded on Maggie's motto "empower the patient" through a "self-help" strategy, improves people's wellbeing during treatment and recovery (Maggie's Evidence, 2015) to the point that we can speak of the therapeutic power of the Maggie's centre.

The Maggie's centre was conceived by Maggie and Charles Jencks—both designers and landscape architects—as a reaction to Maggie's experience lived when she was diagnosed with terminal cancer at Edinburgh hospital in 1994. To counteract the depressing conditions of the hospital environment, as well as the depersonalising treatment they had received, the Jencks worked for 18 months, during which Maggie managed to outlast her diagnosis of "two to three months to live". The goal was to create a welcoming and familiar environment, a non-clinical and anti-institutional environment that offered people with cancer—and their families and their friends—the "many things" that Maggie wanted for them. Born on the remains of a derelict building on the edge of the hospital grounds that had been reclaimed and repurposed, since it was inaugurated in 1996, the Maggie's centre has hardly changed and, as described by Jencks in his book *The Architecture of Hope*, over time has strengthened in its 'hybrid' nature of four types brought together in a 'whole': "A hospital that is not an institution, a house that is not a home, a religious retreat that is not denominational, a place of art that is not a museum" (Jencks, 2015, p. 7).

As its main feature, the Maggie's centre is a healthcare building that does not look like one. Generally located next to the hospital's Oncology Unit, on a land donated or leased by the National Health Service (NHS) that was once a car park or abandoned area, the iconic and seductive or, conversely, hidden and intriguing Maggie's centre welcomes here—now a lush garden—people with cancer, their families and friends, all equally considered "visitors". Once through the door, newcomers are warmly greeted by the staff, invited to take a seat in the welcome area or in the library, and reassured of their concerns with a cup of tea. Without reception desks, plaques on doors or badges on uniforms, the domestic environment devoid of signs of sanitary architecture—where 'sanitary', as used in this book, is a term that derives from the Latin *sanus* (=healthy), which refers to conditions affecting hygiene and health (Glosbe Dictionary, 2023)—helps staff support visitors by establishing an informal relationship from the outset, in which the building is considered a "member of the staff". At this juncture, the combination of a bright entrance, a quiet and familiar atmosphere and an open layout that directly overlooks the large kitchen, generates a strong emotional state in people that often makes them say, through tears: "I don't know why I'm doing this", "I can't explain it". With the help of the staff, after a few moments, people take a long sigh and feel a sense of relief enhanced by the fact that, unlike at the hospital where the first thing they ask you is to fill in forms, at Maggie's people walk in without having to declare who they are or where they come from, which makes them feel safe.

As a first impact on users, this feature makes people with cancer feel like normal people who can freely express their emotions and feelings. Embedded in the kitchen table or 'kitchenism'—a serious joke coined by Charles Jencks that expresses informality and good humour—Maggie's normality allows people to find the best way to feel at ease and to decide at will if and when to fully commit to the centre, leaving them free to leave at any time.

> All the buildings taken as a group are colourful and basically upbeat: the war on cancer is not the primary note they strike. Their domesticity and slightly unusual shape suggest that they might be the friendly clubhouse of an obscure religious sect dedicated to golf. However, the metaphor of 'normality' (which some people may have problems seeing as a rhetorical trope) is also very strong. Tea and cushions – 'kitchenism' – are the recurrent keynote. It displaces the fact of cancer from the exotic and horrific into the everyday and accepted.
>
> (Jencks and Heathcote, 2010, p. 34)

While sharing the same ingredients, the other characteristic of Maggie's centres is that they are all different from each other. This variety comes from the different sites they sit on, but above all from the free interpretation left to the architects of the Architectural Brief, the official set of instructions that architects receive when asked to design their centre (Appendix I). Written upon Maggie Keswick's wishes and ideas soon after her death, the Brief is the essence of Maggie's philosophy that has remained almost unchanged over time—with small additions in 2003 and 2007—becoming the current Maggie's Architecture and Landscape Brief (2015). Unlike any other brief, the concise Brief does not prescribe technical solutions but requires beauty and values through diversified types of space that allow centre users to experience a variety of feelings. Based on the belief that "design is a form of care", the Architectural Brief governs the triangular relationship—what I call Maggie's Triad—in which Maggie's co-clients and the architect work together to benefit the users.

Although Maggie could not see it realised, due to her death in 1995, thanks to Charles Jencks, Laura Lee and Marcia Blakenham—respectively Maggie's oncological nurse and Maggie's best friend—Maggie's Edinburgh (1996) quickly gained visibility despite, as its architect Richard Murphy said, no one initially thought that the project would be replicated with such success in the UK and abroad. Today, Maggie's organisation has grown and strengthened into a vast network of people and centres (Appendix III) that welcome over 290,000 people every year (Maggie's Volunteer Handbook, 2020). Regardless of this breadth, in this book I want to concentrate on the seed that transformed "a small stable building within the hospital grounds into a flexible space from which the centre could operate" (Blakenham, 2007, p. 3). Precisely for this reason, the focus of the book is the essence of Maggie's original model and not the proliferation of its many centres, even if this fact—its reiteration—confirms the power of its replicable model. In architecture, when a model, whose essential aspects remain solid while evolving and subtly transforming over time, is repeatable, it means defining a type or an archetype (Martí Aris, 2021).

Healing vs. Therapeutic

The meaning of the term 'healing' with respect to 'therapeutic' is quite substantial. Although the Cambridge Dictionary (2023a, 2023b) describes both of them as 'curative' and, in current usage, people regard them as interchangeable, conventionally the former has physical/medical references ("process of becoming well again, especially after a cut or other injury"), while the second is mainly psychological ("making someone feel happier and more relaxed or healthier") applicable to any situation that aims to "increase the wellbeing" of people. The real difference, however, lies in their etymology and in the subject of reference: 'healing', derived from the Old English hǣlan (*hal*=whole) that means 'to make sound or whole' (Merriam-Webster, 2023a), is considered to refer to the sick person, while 'therapeutic', derived from the ancient Greek ϑεραπευτικός (*therapeutikós*) (*therapeuein*=to attend, to care) that means 'inclined to serve, to take care of' (Merriam-Webster, 2023b), is considered to refer to the person who cares.

The interchangeability of the terms is also justified by the fact that once this difference did not exist. From Greek healing temples to monastic infirmaries, the mineral springs in the natural landscape or the medicinal herbs in the *horti conclusi* had both 'healing' and 'therapeutic' purposes by acting on both the body and the mind. Over the centuries, with scientific progress and the loss of the idea that access to nature could be healing or therapeutic, body and mind have split and the machine—and chemistry—has taken the place of nature, whose presence in hospitals has become pure decoration (Cooper Marcus and Barnes, 1999). One day, however, Roger Ulrich (1984) demonstrated that rooms with windows overlooking nature rather than a brick wall provided hospital patients with psychological support that accelerated their physical healing process. Much progress has been made since then and today, in the hospital setting, we can speak of 'healing architecture' when a healthcare environment interacts with nature (even adopting virtual solutions), stimulates the senses with natural materials and colours and is free from environmental stressors such as noise, glare, poor air quality and lack of privacy (Ulrich & Zimring, 2004).

The best historical reference for both 'healing' and 'therapeutic' architecture, to this day, remains that of the healing temples of Asclepius, holistic complexes of sophisticated architecture immersed in splendid landscapes where, for almost ten centuries during the Hellenistic and Roman period (V B.C.–IV A.D.), the Ancient Greeks offered therapies to the sick by practicing the medicine of the mythological God. Among the more than 300 built, the one of Epidaurus—which Maggie and Charles visited in the 1970s—was the most famous therapeutic centre in the classical world. Besides the *Asclepeion*, the temple dedicated to Asclepius, the sanctuary included the *abaton* or sacred dormitory for the sick, the *katagòghion* where family members accompanying the sick were welcomed, the gymnasium, the stadium, the common baths and the theatre (Torelli, 2005; Christopoulou-Aletra, Togia and Varlami, 2009) (Figure 1.1).

In addition to architecture, the holistic approach was applied to the healing practice, which combined medical care with psychological support. "Here was an integrated system of healthcare which attended to patients as whole person: body, mind, soul, and spirit" (Kearney, 2009, p. xxii). In considering the psychological and emotional aspects, as well as the innate healing mechanisms of every human being, fundamental for the healing procedure (Christopoulou-Aletra et al., 2009), what has guided the whole of Western medicine, from Asclepius and Hippocrates onwards, was the 'mind-as-important-as-the-body' concept. But, as neuroscientist Antonio Damasio explains in his book *Descartes' Error* (1994), it was René Descartes (1596–1650) who, by separating the mind from the body, changed the course of medicine and history.

> So that this "me", that is to say, the soul by which I am what I am, is entirely distinct from body, and is even more easy to know than is the latter; and even if body were not, the soul would not cease to be what it is.
>
> (Descartes, 1637, quoted by Damasio, 1994, p. 249)

By separating the mind (*psyché*)—soul for Christianity—from the body (*soma*), Descartes has in fact also separated Architecture from Medicine—or Health—eradicating the idea that a physical and social environment can affect the wellbeing of the body that will impact that of the mind. In antiquity, the cosmos was a metaphor of harmony and perfection for both Architecture and Medicine. What unites these two disciplines, born simultaneously in ancient Egypt, in 2800 B.C., under Imhotep—a deified architect known not for his architecture but for his health practice—is their orientation to the future. Both professions are hope-oriented and share the ideal for a better future, a future that changes (Jencks, 2017). As Esther Sternberg writes in her book *Healing Spaces* (2009):

> There is a turning point in the course of healing when you go from the dark side to the light, when your interest in the world revives and where despair gives way to hope. And you lie in bed, you suddenly notice the dappled sunlight on the blinds and no longer turn your head and shield your eyes. (…) This is the point when destructive forces of illness give way to healing. In every sense, it is a turning point – a turning of your mind's awareness from a focus on your inner self to a focus on the outer world. Physicians and nurses know that a patient's sudden interest in external things is the first sign that healing has begun.
>
> (Sternberg, 2009, p. 1)

If hospitals heal by acting on the body and allowing patients to move towards the 'turning point', other healthcare facilities or any architecture can potentially be therapeutic by acting on the mind and soul, which will consequently help the

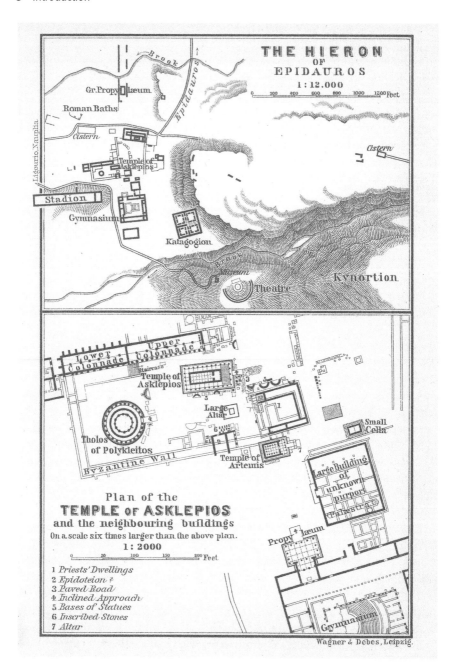

FIGURE 1.1 EPIDAURUS/EPIDAVROS. Hieron Asklepios/Asklepius temple/sanctuary plans 1909 map (Purchased by © 2020 Antiqua Print Gallery Ltd).

body react. This is the case of the non-clinical Maggie's centre, where the sensory architecture combined with the offer of psychological support are essential to start the therapeutic process as "a product of the human mind and of material circumstances" (Gesler, 1992, p. 743). Reminding the reader that traditionally, "pain and disease have been inspiring art and architecture", this book also aims to reunite 'therapeutic' with 'architecture', "an intimate cocktail, the necessary relationship between the social and the physical, the spiritual and the painful, the service and the architectural setting" (Jencks, 2015, pp. 13–14).

Towards a Construction of Health

At the end of the nineteenth century, to facilitate the healing process, all hospitals had large windows and skylights exposed to the sun. This idea was born from the founder of modern nursing, Florence Nightingale who, dedicating herself to the care of the sick, was revolutionary in the belief that sunlit rooms were healthy while dark rooms were harmful. Almost a 100 years later, in 1948, the NHS represented a new revolutionary moment for British healthcare: healthcare was to be "universal, comprehensive and free" (Gorsky, 2008, p. 438). To this end, public health institutions, from large urban hospitals to small rural clinics, were concentrated in a single system characterised by a single architectural language.

To demonstrate the 'healthiness' of the architecture, the NHS architects chose the 'podium + tower' model, i.e. an urban volume accessible to the public on the ground floor and, for hygienic reasons, the ward tower above, applying it to all hospitals in Great Britain. The first notable building of this type was the Princess Margaret Hospital in Swindon, designed by Powell & Moya, opened in 1966 and demolished in 2004. Soon adopted throughout Europe, the British model, which provided natural light and panoramic views, was intended to be the NHS charity manifesto. Despite the noble intention, however, this trend almost immediately changed course becoming a demonstration, through architecture of the power of the healthcare system. Influenced by Taylorism theories and a belief in scientific research, NHS architects began designing large repetitive buildings which resulted in the construction of dehumanised hospitals (Jencks, 2015).

In an attempt to counteract this rampant trend, as Richard Murphy explained to me, in the 1970s there was a reaction. The British economist Ernst Friedrich Schumacher coined the slogan "Small Is Beautiful" (1973), which helped support Ted Cullinan's project for a small cottage hospital in Lambeth (1976).

> It was a very beautiful building, and it was basically a GPs surgery, a sort of information centre. I think there were about 20 beds and a garden, and it was the sort of reassertion of human hospital scale, actually. But then Mrs. Thatcher said: 'Let's go big again'.
>
> (*Murphy, 01.06.2018*)

As a result, hospitals in the UK started to grow again along with scientific advances, which, despite leading cancer patients to survive longer (NHS, 2020), have seen an increase in the rate of diagnoses. "Currently one in two of us born after 1960 will be diagnosed with cancer at some point in our lives" (UK Government, 2019). In the UK this means that the gigantism of hospitals will not stop, on the contrary, hospitals will get even bigger. Addressing architects who work in healthcare, but also in architecture in general, Sternberg therefore asks: "Can we design places so as to enhance their healing properties?" (2009, p. 1).

Today, architects who recognise the importance of ensuring a positive experience for their users answer this question by adopting so-called 'sensory architecture'. However, in the UK, healthcare architects have not yet adopted this design approach despite the good examples existing in the world and the vast literature on the subject, which ultimately highlights the discrepancy between the ideal world of theory and the functional world of practice dictated by the 'Constructor of Health'. Considered a field of action for "specialists", who do not like ideas or changes, as we will see in Chapter 7, the architecture of hospitals is still tied to a functionalistic logic and depersonalised design.

> They like to do things their own way, with no culture and ambition for beauty, but with a lot of knowledge of fast realisation and gain.
>
> (*de Rijke, 17.12.2018*)

According to Alex de Rijke—who had an indirect negative experience with the NHS—anyone who enters a hospital today certainly does not have the impression that architecture and design are a priority, but only understands that treatment is disguised as a mechanistic system. Even for Ellen van Loon (OMA), the second architect I interviewed, the depersonalisation of spaces has now become unacceptable.

> When we visited Glasgow, the state of the Queen Elizabeth University Hospital was so inhuman that it was like going to a factory, where you are treated like a number on a list – patient number 3 out of 65. As an alternative, we started wondering how a person would prefer to be treated.
>
> (*van Loon, 15.05.2018*)

On the contrary, whoever enters a Maggie's centre immediately receives the clear message that "design is a form of care" and that the human dimension is central, highlighted by the way the staff expresses total dedication to visitors, suggesting that Maggie's focus is the care of the person.

> Maggie's starts with the person, with the visitor, and everything we do rolls out from the relationship we developed with our architect as well as the relationship

that we develop with our construction team starts with that principle. Everybody has to understand that that person, that visitor is the most important thing and that they are our product.

(*Maggie's@Salus, 2021*)

With the simple question "Could things be different?" the "Maggie's Centres Movement", as Charles Jencks (2005) called it at the time, is in fact challenging the traditional mechanistic and unsightly view of public health, promoting instead an approach that is centred on the person and his/her fundamental need for beauty and values. In this provocation, in addition to physical opposition, Maggie's is also a cultural challenge, asking the NHS to react to the *status quo* of the healthcare environment as a whole. By activating the change that will lead to the "Construction of Health", as we will see better in Chapter 7, Maggie's represents a model to be applied to other health and non-health facilities and, perhaps, also to architecture in general. In this construction, Maggie's model could initiate a system of cooperation in which all the structures supporting people's physical and psychological care could collaborate with the hospital and with each other. Adhering to the goal that calls for "integration" according to Jencks' will, and in line with Maggie's belief that "design is a form of care", hospitals and other organisations will look at Maggie's not only for the ability to entrust an active role for the patient, but also for the architectural metaphor of iconic joy (Jencks, 2015), which has begun to interest more and more people in the healthcare world.

Phenomenology, Neuroscience and Architecture

As anticipated in the Preface, in an attempt to experience first-hand what visitors feel in a Maggie's centre and understand the source of their wellbeing, in my PhD ethnographic work I immersed myself for nearly four months in three centres adopting phenomenology, the method for investigating the structure of our lived experience in the world formulated by Edmund Husserl (1982 [1913]).

Mathematician by training, averse to the psychologism of the early twentieth century which claimed to have an objective knowledge of the objects of reality, Husserl (1859–1938) argued that we can understand the objects we encounter in our experience only by not separating them from the way in which they appear to the subject (Held, 2003). Lived in the first person, always oriented towards something, this experience is acted upon by the *intentionality* of consciousness and is effective through the encounter with objects which, as Husserl says, are "things" that must be approached by suspending any preconception or prejudice (1982 [1913]). In this encounter of the 'subject' with the 'object', the subject is limited by the partial vision of the object and feels emotions emerge due to the excess of expectation: not appearing in full, the non-visible part of the object leaves room for the imagination, making us live an emotional experience that goes beyond what is visible (Husserl, 1989 [1913]).

Influenced by Husserl, from whom however he departs in regards the Cartesian consciousness–body dichotomy, Marcel Merleau-Ponty (1908–1961) tells us that the perceiving subject is no longer a consciousness located inside a body, but the body itself is the means of experience. In his book *Phenomenology of Perception* (2012 [1945]), Merleau-Ponty describes how, going beyond the five senses, the perceptual experience involves the whole body and how the body acts as an interface between the individual's inner world and the external social world (Hale, 2017). In order for the body to perceive, it must move, because if it does not move it cannot experience and the world cannot appear. The process of exploration and discovery, which impacts our experiences, is our way of understanding the world.

In a Maggie's centre, architecture invites people to be part of the space and, thanks to 'spatial interaction rather than walls', to move and interact with others. By recognising the emotions and thoughts of others, people see the other 'as one of them', or them 'as part of the others', giving rise to *intersubjectivity* which, together with *empathy,* are basic concepts of phenomenology (Zahavi, 2001). Within the space consequently, there is no *ipse* or separate entity that refers to other subjects, but rather a relational structure in which the different subjectivities are immersed from the very beginning (Merleau-Ponty, 1949–1952, cited in Spina, 2014). This leads us to affirm that subjectivity always presupposes a relationship and that, only when the subject feels the need for a human relationship, does it become such: subjects break their isolation to enter and give themselves to others (Basaglia, 1981).

Intersubjectivity and *empathy* are also among the main objectives of contemporary research in cognitive neuroscience, "that is, that branch of neuroscience that has as its object of study the more sophisticated aspects of our intelligent behaviour" (Gallese, 2009, p. 1*).

> We could say that one of the fundamental questions that Edmund Husserl (1859–1938), father of phenomenology, had tried to answer, today can be done precisely by cognitive neuroscience: how is it possible to study subjectivity, the first-person approach to reality, so as to be able to scientifically describe it without limiting oneself to understanding it in the ineffable way of introspection, which does not allow for the objective communication typical of science?
>
> (Gallese, 2009, p. 2*)

The answer to this question comes from the interdisciplinarity between humanistic and scientific culture. In architecture, this had already been intuited by Richard Neutra (1954) who had argued that, in order to survive, design should have approached biological sciences. Precisely with this intent, in the 1960s, at MIT, the term "Neuroscience" was coined which, in an interdisciplinary way and involving scientists from different backgrounds, aimed to study the brain in relation to the built or natural environment. In the same years, the biologist Jonas Salk—who succeeded in discovering the polio vaccine thanks to an illuminating experience derived from a visit to the Basilica of San Francesco d'Assisi, proving evidence of the connection between the environment and cognitive abilities—founded the Salk Institute for Biological Studies with the aim of inspiring more and more scientists. Among the most beautiful buildings designed by Louis Khan (1963), the Salk Institute in San Diego is now home to the Academy of Neuroscience for Architecture (ANFA) which, together with the Neuroscience Applied to Architectural Design (NAAD) master's programme of the Università Iuav di Venezia, promotes at an academic level the interdisciplinarity between neuroscience and architecture, better known as 'Neuroarchitecture' which, according to many, is now essential.

Maggie's architects are also close to this belief as they know that by acting on the body and mind, influencing the conditions of calm, tension and self-confidence, an environment can be fundamental. "Architecture is an art that has the power to arouse emotions" (*McVoy, 05.26.2018*). At Maggie's, emotions and feelings are deliberately generated by the architecture whose spatiality, at first, makes one say "I don't know what it is", "I don't know how to explain it" and, then, helps to regain self-confidence and control. According to Damasio (1994), emotional state influences decision-making, explaining why at Maggie's people with cancer are facilitated in taking action.

> In some circumstances, too much thinking may be far less advantageous than no thinking at all. (…) [Emotion] allows the possibility of making living beings act smartly without having to think smartly (…) and a good thing too: we have discovered that the emotions alone can solve many–but not all–the problems posed by our complex environment.
>
> (Damasio, 1994, p. xvii)

As John Paul Eberhard, founder of ANFA (2002), explains, architects and neuroscientists use the brain and mind in a very similar way. However, the link between architectural design and knowledge of neuroscience is still very weak, because the conscious process of modeling this context is only partially understood by architects and most neuroscientists think of architecture as a profession dealing with aesthetics (Eberhard, 2007). Indeed, today's architects are not always aware of this potential and, not knowing the biology of the person—which explains how the brain and the body together perceive the world through the senses and their receptors and act on it through movement and voice—cannot predict how people respond to the environment. As Damasio (1994) explains:

> Neuroanatomy is the fundamental discipline in neuroscience, from the level of microscopic single neurons (nerve cells) to that of the macroscopic systems spanning the entire brain. There can be no hope of understanding the many levels of brain function if we do not have a detailed knowledge of brain geography at multiple scales.
>
> (Damasio, 1994, p. 25)

Without expecting architects to delve into the subject to such an extent, it is true however that the first noteworthy series of drawings in history, the treatise on neuro-anatomy *Cerebri Anatome* (1663) by the physiologist Sir Thomas Willis, was illustrated by Christopher Wren, the architect of St. Paul's Cathedral in London. Driven by this revelation (Sternberg, 2009), I went to the Royal Society of Medicine in London to look at the book and was struck by how the anatomical drawings—whose accuracy due to "the most illustrious man, Dr. Wren, [who] for his extraordinary humanity, was not burdened with drawing the most numerous figures of the Brain and Skull, so that the works were more exact, with his most skilled hands" (Willis, 1663)—were not so different from those of the *Quattro Libri dell'Architettura* (1570) by Andrea Palladio who, as remembered in the film "Palladio" (Gatti, 2019), less than a century earlier had represented buildings in section for the first time. Reaffirming, through this collaboration, the link between Architecture and Medicine (or Health) promoted by Charles Jencks, the fact that in the seventeenth century the two professionals of the two disciplines, joining forces, have worked together on the representation of the brain, seems to be the perfect reference for this book which aims to reconnect architecture and health, seen through the lens of neuroscience (Figure 1.2A–1.2D).

The Structure of the Book

After this introduction, which provides key insights for understanding the unconventional nature of the Maggie's centre, proceeding on the "therapeutic" (holistic, emotional) and no longer "healing" (partial, rational) territory, the reader will find six chapters and the epilogue.

Before definitively entering Maggie's world, Chapter 2 recounts my ethnographic work undertaken in three Maggie's centres, where the ability of the building to generate a therapeutic environment based on 'movement', 'hybrid' and 'non-therapeutic/therapeutic nature' emerged. Within 'movement', on a neurological level, the "sense of movement" or *kinesthesia* (Berthoz, 2000)—i.e. the experience of our body moving in response to the environment—is connected to perception, a fact that was proven by the discovery of mirror neurons (Di Pellegrino et al., 1992). The three elements, inherent in Maggie's open space, together bring to life the principle of *flexibility*, which is ultimately the universally recognised attribute of a therapeutic environment. Chapter 3 finally opens the centre's doors to the reader by describing Maggie's components, namely the organisation, the support programme and the building—with its architecture, art, furniture and gardens—which, by interacting with each other, initiate the therapeutic process. Chapter 4 reveals Maggie's fundamentals by reinforcing Jencks' idea that architecture and health are closely related: Maggie's *therapeutikós*, which finds its reference in the ancient Greeks upon which the support programme is based; the Architectural Brief which finds analogies with the Benedictine Rule (549) and in which, like at Maggie's, architecture, programme and values coincide; Maggie's Triad, i.e., as mentioned, the triangular relationship in which co-clients and architects work closely together to design a "superb" product for users.

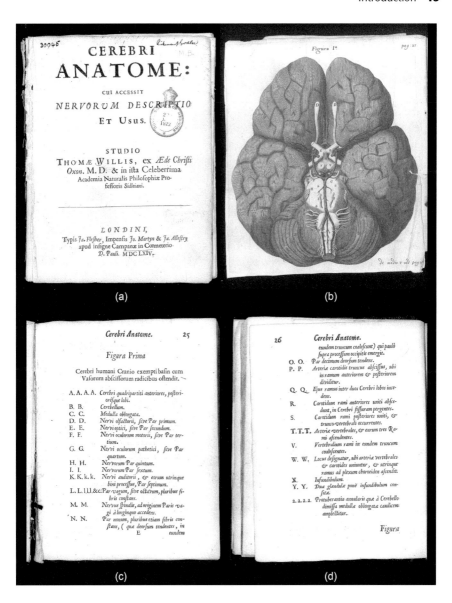

FIGURE 1.2A–1.2D   Thomas Willis' Cerebri Anatome, 1664. Cover page, Sir Christopher Wren's drawing of the base of the brain "with the roots of the vessels cut off", pp. 25–26, *Figura Prima*, legend of the different parts of the brain (Courtesy of The Royal Society of Medicine).

Entering the heart of the Maggie's centre and giving a voice to the users (visitors and staff), Chapter 5 focuses on the synergistic co-operation between the sophisticated architecture (*place*) and Maggie's users (*people*), giving life to Maggie's Synergy. Within this synergy, which allows for the psychological flexibility of the visitors, the five-step healing process is clarified, explaining how people move from a state of shock to a state of stability. Having observed that in the various centres people talk and behave in the same way, it emerges that what connects people and buildings, even distant ones, is the open space that triggers empathy, a sort of 'emotional imitation'. Unveiling Maggie's Phenomenology, Chapter 6 clarifies what exactly in architecture generates its 'experiential field', i.e. what Merleau-Ponty (1945–2012) called the "space of experience" or "phenomenal field", the one loaded with forces that push and move people's bodies and make them say "I don't know what it is", "I don't know how to explain it". By feeling active and not passive and living an 'embodied experience', people finally recognise the therapeutic power of the Maggie's centre. Based on Maggie's ability to become a 'unique', yet 'repeatable' model, finally, Chapter 7 proposes a paradigm shift in the Architecture of Care and recommends the Maggie's centre as an emerging paradigm for future healthcare and non-healthcare facilities.

In a paradigmatic logic, if an 'embodied spatial experience' is essential to tolerate traumatic transitions in the healthcare sector, it must also be so in architecture in general, since finding *wellbeing* is the priority of all human beings. Learning from its users that the Maggie's centre produces therapeutic effects and a taxonomy of feelings, the book's epilogue suggests a new way of perceiving and cataloguing architecture, which will no longer be by typology or function, but will arise from the interaction between the effects released by the building and the emotions and feelings generated in people. While not measurable with certainty, it is my growing conviction that this way of judging a building, in addition to attempting to re-unite 'mind' and 'body' and 'architecture' and 'health', can help architecture rediscover its human values and people to think more about their own response towards the built environment which, being culturally and experientially determined, can always aspire to improve.

References

Alice Dousova- Zuketa LTD (2023) The Cosmic House. link https://vimeo.com/641891654/dba89579ff

Basaglia, F. (1981) *Scritti I, 1953–1968. Dalla psichiatria fenomenologica all'esperienza di Gorizia.* Torino: Einaudi

Berthoz, A. (2000) *The Brain's Sense of Movement.* Boston: Harvard University Press

Blakenham, M. (2007) 'Foreword and Maggie's Centres: Marching on', in Keswick, M. (1994) *A View from the Front Line.* https://maggies-staging.s3.amazonaws.com/media/filer_public/5b/f6/5bf6f8c7-37e4-4b0a-b09d-6ad48d66387d/view-from-the-front-line.pdf

Cambridge Dictionary (2023a) 'Definition of Healing'. https://dictionary.cambridge.org/dictionary/english/healing

Cambridge Dictionary (2023b) 'Definition of Therapeutic'. https://dictionary.cambridge.org/dictionary/english/therapeutic

Christopoulou-Aletra, H., Togia, A. and Varlami, C. (2009) *The 'Smart' Asclepieion: A Total Healing Environment*. Department of History of Medicine, Aristotele University of Thessaloniki

Cooper Marcus, C. and Barnes, M. (1999) *Healing Gardens: Therapeutic Benefits and Design Reccomandations*. New York: John Wiley & Sons

Damasio, A. (1994) *Descartes' Error: Emotion, Reason, and the Human Brain*. London: Vintage

Di Pellegrino, G., Fadiga, L., Fogassi, L., Gallese, V. and Rizzolatti, G. (1992) 'Understanding motor events: a neurophysiological study', Experimental Brain Research, Springer-Verlag, 91, pp. 176–180.

Eberhard, J. P. (2007) *Architecture and the Brain: A New Knowledge Base from Neuroscience*. Belmond (IA): Greenway Communications LLC.

Gallese, V. (2009) 'Neuroscienze e fenomenologia', *Treccani Terzo Millennio*, Vol. I, pp. 1–32. https://www.treccani.it/enciclopedia/neuroscienze-e-fenomenologia_%28XXI-Secolo%29/

Gatti (2019) *Palladio*. https://www.youtube.com/watch?v=4p_jiI1PqYc&feature=youtu.be&ab_channel=MAGNITUDOFILM

Gesler, W. M. (1992) 'Therapeutic Landscapes: Medical Issues in Light of the New Cultural Geography', *Social Science & Medicine*, 34(7), pp. 735–746

Glosbe Dictionary (2023) 'Translation of Sanitary'. https://glosbe.com/en/la/sanitary

Gorsky, M. (2008) 'The British National Health Service 1948–2008: A Review of the Historiography', *Social History of Medicine*, (21)3, pp. 437–460

Hale, J. (2017) *Merleau-Ponty for Architects*. London and New York: Routledge

Held, K. (2003) 'Husserl's Phenomenological Method', in Rodemeyer, L. (ed. and transl.) *The New Husserl: A Critical Reader*. Bloomington: Indiana University Press, pp. 3–31

Husserl, E. (1982 [1913]) *Ideas Pertaining to a Pure Phenomenology and to a Phenomenological Philosophy. First Book: General Introduction to a Pure Phenomenology*. Translated by F. Kersten. The Hague: Nijhoff

Husserl, E. (1989 [1913]) *Ideas Pertaining to a Pure Phenomenology and to a Phenomenological Philosophy. Second Book: Studies in the Phenomenology of Constitution*. Translated by Richard Rojcewicz and André Schuwer. Dordrecht: Kluwer Academic

Jencks, C. (2005) 'The Maggie Centres', *Fourth Door Review*, 7, pp. 30–33. http://www.fourthdoor.co.uk/review/issue_7.php

Jencks, C. (2015) *The Architecture of Hope: Maggie's Cancer Caring Centres* (2nd ed.). London: Frances Lincoln

Jencks, C. (2017) 'Maggie's Architecture: The Deep Affinities between Architecture and Health', *Architectural Design*, 87(2), pp. 66–75

Jencks, C. and Heathcote, E. (2010) *The Architecture of Hope: Maggie's Cancer Caring Centres* (1st ed.). London: Frances Lincoln

Kearney, M. (2009) *A Place of Healing: Working with Nature & Soul at the End of Life*. New Orleans: Spring Journal Books

Keswick, M. (1994) *A View From The Frontline*. Revised and reprinted in 2003 and 2007. https://maggies-staging.s3.amazonaws.com/media/filer_public/5b/f6/5bf6f8c7-37e4-4b0a-b09d-6ad48d66387d/view-from-the-front-line.pdf

Maggie's Brief (2015) 'Architectural and Landcape Brief'. https://maggies-staging.s3.amazonaws.com/media/filer_public/e0/3e/e03e8b60-ecc7-4ec7-95a1-18d9f9c4e7c9/maggies_architecturalbrief_2015.pdf

Maggie's Evidence (2015) 'Maggie's Evidence-based_Programme Web Spreads'. https://maggies-staging.s3.amazonaws.com/media/filer_public/78/3e/783ef1ba-cd5b-471c-b04f-1fe25095406d/evidence-based_programme_web_spreads.pdf

Maggie's Volunteer Handbook (2020) https://maggies-staging.s3.amazonaws.com/media/filer_public/4e/cd/4ecdf73c-fef1-430b-aea3-cc50cf62c1ce/maggies_volunteers_handbook_2020.pdf

Martí Arís, C. (2021) *Variation of Identity - Type in Architecture* (transl. by Claudia Mion and Fabio Licitra) Dijon: Les Presses du Réel

Merleau-Ponty, M. (2012 [1945]) *Phenomenology of Perception*. Translated by D. A. Landes. Abington and New York: Routledge

Merriam-Webster (2023a) 'Etymology for Heal'. https://www.merriam-webster.com/dictionary/heal

Merriam-Webster (2023b) 'Etymology for Therapeutic'. https://www.merriam-webster.com/dictionary/therapeutic

NHS (2020) 'The Government's Cancer Reform Strategy'. https://www.england.nhs.uk/publication/nhs-cancer-programme-update-report/

Spina, M. (2014) 'Fenomenologia e scienze umane. Osservazioni a partire dai corsi di psicologia e pedagogia del bambino', in Verardi, D. (ed.) *Lapis. Note E Testi, Psychofenia* - Anno XVII, n. 30/2014, pp. 111–122

Sternberg, E. (2009) *Healing Spaces: The Science of Place and Wellbeing*. Cambridge, MA: Belknap Press of Harvard University Press

Torelli, M. (2005) 'Fenomenologia del culto di Asclepio. I casi di Epidauro, Trezene ed Atene', in De Miro, E., Sfameni Gasparro, G. and Calì, V. (eds.) Il culto di Asclepio nell'area mediterranea. Rome: Giangemi Editore.

Ulrich, R. S. (1984) 'View through a Window May Influence Recovery from Surgery', *Science*, 224(4647), pp. 420–421

Ulrich, R. and Zimring, C. (2004) 'The Role of the Physical Environment in the Hospital of the 21st Century: A Once-in-a-Lifetime Opportunity'. Report to The Center for Health Design for the *Designing the 21st Century Hospital Project*. Robert Wood Johnson Foundation'. https://www.healthdesign.org/system/files/Ulrich_Role%20of%20Physical_2004.pdf

UK Government (2019) 'Office for National Statistics', 26 April. https://blog.ons.gov.uk/2019/04/26/are-there-more-people-diagnosed-with-cancer/#:~:text=Since%202001%2C%20the%20number%20of, some%20point%20in%20our%20lives

Willis, T. (1663) *Cerebri Anatome: cui accessit Nervorum Descriptio et Usus.* Londini: D.Pauli

Zahavi, D. (2001) 'Beyond Empathy. Phenomenological Approaches to Intersubjectivity', *Journal of Consciousness Studies*, 8(5–7), pp. 151–167

2

MAGGIE'S THERAPEUTIC ENVIRONMENT

My Experience Lived in the Maggie's Centre

At the beginning of September 2019, after visiting all the Maggie's centres—where I was able to chat informally with the staff—interviewing 12 Maggie's architects—so I could verify the application of the Architectural Brief to their project—and, finally, having a conversation with Maggie's co-clients—as a cross-check of the information received from the architects—I was ready to live an immersive experience in the three centres assigned to me, Maggie's Dundee (2003), Maggie's Oldham (2017) and Maggie's Barts (2017). The purpose of this new work phase, which lasted until the end of December 2019, was to verify that Howells' postulate—"the synergy between people and place enables psychological flexibility"—was also valid from an architectural point of view. Ultimately, I wanted to discover what it is in the Maggie's centre that generates therapeutic effects in users, i.e. the link between the design methodology adopted by the architects and the flexible mental state enabled in Maggie's users; more precisely, I wanted to understand how this link is able to establish an effective therapeutic environment.

Just to give the reader an idea of the context in which I was about to operate, I will quickly describe the three centres, all enriched by a very strong symbolic value. Maggie's Dundee, for example, conceived as a 'strange' white Scottish cottage with a 'lighthouse'—which represents a beacon of hope—stands out on the edge of a large green plain, where a labyrinth carved inside symbolises our life's journey. Maggie's Oldham, thought as 'a box with a hole' and 'a tree in it'—a symbol of life—and a boundless view of the Pennine hills, stands above the site of a former mortuary—now a garden open to the entire hospital—inspired by the Chinese stilt house, guaranteeing safety and foresight. Finally, Maggie's Barts, conceived as 'a large translucent glass case' dotted with colours—inspired by the

DOI: 10.4324/9781003244516-2

coloured notations of medieval music found in the nearby church of Saint Bartholomew the Great (XII AD)—is placed discreetly in the corner of the courtyard of the historic hospital in London, becoming a 'lantern' illuminating people's path in the dark (Figures 2.1–2.3).

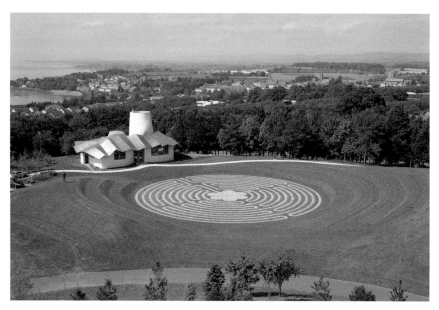

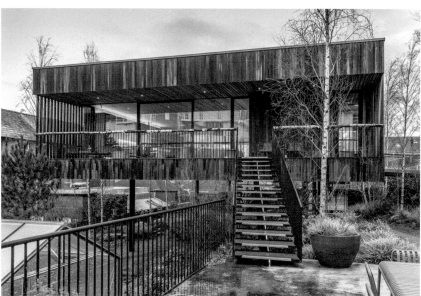

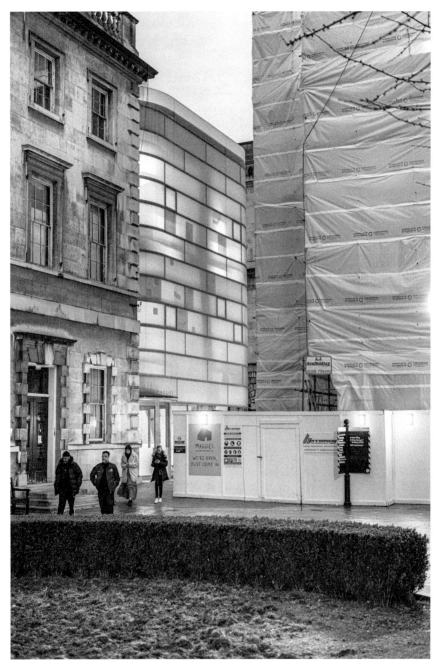

FIGURES 2.1–2.3   Maggie's Dundee (2003) (Courtesy of Maggie's), Maggie's Oldham (2017) and Maggie's Barts (2017) (©Marco Castelli Nirmal). During the day Maggie's buildings invite you to enter; at night, like lanterns, they illuminate the path of people in the darkness.

As already mentioned in the introduction, the flexible state of mind enabled in Maggie's users comes from the message contained in the quote by Maggie Keswick Jencks: "Above all, what matters is not to lose the joy of living for fear of dying" (1994). Founded by Steven Hayes (Hayes and Smith, 2005)—one of the fathers of ACT (Acceptance and Commitment Therapy)—to help people respond to negative life events by offering them a way of behaving, Psychological Flexibility has affinities with ancient Asclepian healing. In his book *A Place of Healing* (Kearney, 2009), Michael Kearney comes very close to the concept of psychological flexibility when he reveals that Asclepian healing (V B.C.–IV A.D.) resides in suffering, allowing "that person to find a way of living with, and perhaps in time opening more to, the depth of his or her experience" rather than seeking "life as it was before" (2009, p. 47), and perhaps finding healing even if they could not be cured. As we will see in Chapter 4, according to Kearney, therapeutic flexibility may also have created the feeling that the articulated environment was a significant factor in health.

As Lesley Howells explains in her TEDxTalk (Howells, 2016), it is the synergy between the bespoke architecture of the Maggie's centre combined in a vibrant 'fluid dance' with the people within it that enables the concept of psychological flexibility. This state of mind encourages people to open up to moving with the reality of the disease rather than struggling against it, "finding freedom in the choice we are offered" (Howells, 2016). This freedom is added to that given by the architecture of the building that tells its users that "Maggie's is their home and that they are in charge" (*Lee, 16.10.2019*), which leads us to conclude that:

> A therapeutic environment is the meeting point between building and people, and if the building is designed in a particular way, this environment is able to transfer energy to people.
>
> (*Howells, 13.03.2019*)

Starting from this assumption and from the studies on the Maggie's centre by Butterfield and Martin (2014, 2016), Martin (2014, 2016, 2017) and Martin, Nettleton and Buse (2019)—who had attributed the therapeutic nature of the building to the excellence of the artefact, the harmony with which the daily spaces of Maggie's kitchen and her large table (on which 'the illness is placed at the centre') are orchestrated and the synergistic action of "generators of architectural atmospheres", i.e. the combination of materials, light, colour and shape of the buildings together with the good care of the staff—aware that I was about to enter an environment where the psychological impact is very high, I started my preparation. To make sure I would understand the point of view of Maggie's users, but above all, that I would fully live their sensory experience, as mentioned, I opted for a phenomenological and therefore subjective approach, with a perspective no longer of the researcher or architect but rather of the user; furthermore, to have an open and broad perspective, I chose to use four methods of investigation (two of which are discussed in this chapter and two in Chapter 5) with a final follow-up discussion with the participants interested in giving me their opinion on my research and with whom I shared my observations. This multiple methodology had to take into account the fact that, in order to allow for the activities included in the centre's timetable to be carried out, during the day the staff continuously moves the furniture to make a different use of the space, bringing about a change of scenery, explaining why Lesley Howells says:

> We constantly roll up the carpet and then unroll it as we change the background for each of our courses and workshops. And that flexibility, that 'bending' with our environment is what we hope will shape those around us.
>
> (Howells, 2016, 15:50)

Adopting a phenomenological approach meant combining a perspective view with an 'embodied experience'—that is, as I will explain better in Chapter 6, not only that of observing, but also of living the space with the whole body—dynamically participating in the life of the centre. By choosing to immerse myself in Maggie's reality, the fact of not being a person with cancer theoretically ruled out any danger of being incorporated into a cancer-oriented environment and any influence that would ensue. However, because Maggie's intention is to get people involved very quickly, despite my attempts to maintain a position of *super-partes* researcher, as a person I was happy to be engaged not only as an observer/participant in the activities, but also as a confidant of many stories that have marked my life emotionally becoming the starting point of beautiful friendships that continue to this day.

My first method was 'while I participated, I observed'. Trying to understand how the spaces in the centre were used, detect the types of people's movements and identify the most 'therapeutic' areas of the centre, as a participant in social activities, since my work was focused on architecture and people's wellbeing, I participated in those that aimed at 'distracting from cancer' (yoga, Tai chi, expressive art therapy, gentle movement, move-dance-feel, chorus, nutrition, relaxation, sleep soundly) and not in those 'dealing with cancer' (cancer network groups, FSG support groups, 'where now'). During breaks, in the kitchen, I chatted with people, made cups of tea and sometimes helped unload the dishwasher. In quiet hours I would sit and talk to visitors about my research or, on my own, observe the scene taking into account the number of people in the building, their mood (joyful and outgoing or quiet and introverted) and the type of activity performed on that day. In this overview, I also observed those who were simply present without participating in the activities. The final result was a colour map of the different rooms describing the level of "therapeuticity" of the Maggie's centre within the parameters of 'social interaction', 'privacy' and 'counseling', which are the three main purposes of Maggie's programme (Frisone, 2021).

My second method was a mobile method, the 'Move-along', a variation I made of the 'Walk-along' (Rose, Degen and Basdas, 2010), already a combination of the mobile interview of the 'Go-along' (Kusenbach, 2003) with the photo-diary/photo-interview (Latham, 2003). This method—which consisted of following participants on their daily errands and asking them to take pictures of the environment (a shopping mall), download the photos to a laptop, and comment on them in a follow-up interview—aimed to identify the places preferred by users, i.e. how the building generates individual 'affects' and responds to people's expectations and also to understand if such places aroused common impressions. Since Maggie's visitors usually lead a quiet life inside the centre and this method could not be applied, my Move-along became a sort of personalised 'architectural tour' led by those participants who, happy to show me the building, would let me see it through their eyes. In it, speed of movement and pauses were established by them: if the participants entered a room and decided to sit down, I did the same; and if they decided not to continue, but to describe the space while sitting, I humoured them. The 'Sit-along', as I have called this methodological variation, was possible thanks to the open space that allows to see through, even from afar, and the way in which the building solicits a photographic memory in the participants, who were able to describe in detail areas we couldn't see. Although the 'Sit-along' did not involve movement and therefore a phenomenological 'movement-in-the-world', just sitting down and talking to the people who have a daily relationship with the building allowed me to get very close to their experience.

The choice of the 'Move-along'—by the way, made intuitively long before starting my ethnographic work—revealed that 'movement' was the *trait d'union* between me and my participants, the key to accessing people's feelings and the link between the architecture that had generated such feelings and the flexible mental state enabled in Maggie's users. This realisation came a few months after completing my ethnographic work, and in the following chapters, I will explain how I discovered it and what in a Maggie's centre triggers it. I had realised that everything inside the building concurred to create movement: the staff who constantly modify the space to adapt it to new activities with the "constantly roll up the carpet and then unroll it"; Maggie's philosophy that encourages the 'do it yourself' and keeps visitors in action; the architecture that invites you to walk in its open and continuous spaces. Thinking back to the scenes of daily life in the centres, I suddenly understood that, in a Maggie's centre, the body is sensorially captured by the architecture and stimulated by the staff to access anywhere in the building, which generates an active state in Maggie's visitors, the exact opposite of the passive state that occurs in the patient in the hospital.

However, the factor that most convinced me that it was 'movement' that linked the design methodology to psychological flexibility was seeing the photographs on my laptop during the follow-up interview with the 'Move-along' participants. Aiming to investigate what had generated the preferences and affects released by the building in them, the commented review of the photos showed that the participants' experience had been 'embodied', that is, as mentioned, a multisensory experience that involves perception beyond the five senses and that makes the moving body become 'part' of the space, evident in the constant change of points of view of the photographs. By focusing on the impressions generated by their movement in the open and continuous space and what they had felt, the participants were then able to realign their thoughts and describe the therapeutic effects they had experienced. Furthermore, through shots of details such as light sources, shadows, reflections and colours, unexpectedly, the photographic review made me aware of further conditions that the naked eye in motion had not grasped (but the brain did) and that is where the emotions and feelings experienced by individuals immersed in the space of a Maggie's centre originate (Frisone, 2021).

The Three Elements of the Therapeutic Environment

After discovering that 'movement' is the key element that enables *flexibility* and links architecture to psychological flexibility, becoming the first element defining a therapeutic environment, I wanted to find out what other possible clues I could use to define the Maggie's centre as such. Starting from the analysis made under the different aspects that characterise it, which made me understand that 'movement' has a multifaceted nature, I returned to Jencks' "hybrid power" inherent in the Maggie's centre, a hybrid of four types and their opposites: "Each centre is like a house that is not a home, an existentialist religious retreat that is non-denominational, a hospital that is a non-institution, and a place of art that is a non-museum" (Jencks, 2015, p. 7). By examining the characteristics of 'ambiguity' and 'transformation' of the hybrid, as well as its properties of adaptability and reinvention in evolution, I discovered that these attributes lead to psychological wellbeing, thus deciding to elect it as the second element of the therapeutic environment.

Yet, as Maggie's therapeutic nature unfolded, more questions arose. If 'movement' helps to be 'flexible' and 'hybrid' is what defines the 'whole' made of 'many things', and if the Maggie's centre as a 'flexible whole' is a 'therapeutic environment', then the latter should be the result of the application of some kind of scientific knowledge in this field. But what do Maggie's architects know about healing architecture? Were they chosen because they were all specialised in the design of a sanitary building? The answer is NO. None of the 12 architects interviewed had any scientific knowledge of healing architecture. And not only do the architects refuse to think of their Maggie's centre as healing architecture, but, as we saw in the introduction, even the co-clients do not accept this interpretation. And obviously Charles Jencks also never wanted to define the Maggie's centre as a place of healing, but rather as "many things", a hybrid, in fact. However, precisely those feelings of encouragement and action that arise in people thanks to a normal environment devoid of signs of sanitary architecture are the expression of the healing condition of the building. Coming full circle, the paradoxical and enigmatic 'non-therapeutic/therapeutic' nature was revealed as the third element that identifies the Maggie's centre as an effective therapeutic environment.

Movement

As the first element characterising the therapeutic environment of the Maggie's centre, as already seen in the Introduction with Merleau-Ponty (2012 [1945]), 'movement' is our means of perceiving the world. Intended as a catalyst for an active sequence of experiences, at Maggie's movement gives life to daily social life which becomes a real performance, to physical activities which imply constant movement, a 'fluid dance', to the motility in open and continuous spaces of people with 'motor manifestations considered independent of psychic activity'. As neuroscience teaches us, movement stimulates perception, which is the process by which the brain serves to predict future action. By developing a "sense of movement" or *Kinesthesia,* which is our natural activation of several cooperating sensors that prompt the brain to reconstruct movement in the body and in the environment

(Berthoz, 2000), Maggie's visitors, immersed in space, feel active and not passive, a *sine qua non* condition for being able to experience emotions and feelings.

Movement as 'Performativity'

The Maggie's centre, flexible and open to any interpretation, leaves people room for action and gives them the opportunity to situate themselves. During their daily social performance, constantly changing scenarios, buildings and staff contribute to build the background of Maggie's performativity, an open stage that engages users and makes everyone feel valued. According to her concept of performativity, the American feminist and gender theorist and philosopher Judith Butler explains that people come to believe they realise a reality through repetition of words or gestures just like actors playing a script (Butler, 1993). Inside the theatrical space of the Maggie's centre, through the repetition of phrases like 'would you like a cup of tea?' and acts like sitting around the kitchen table, visitors and staff become actors and recite a familiar script, surprisingly encouraging people with cancer to open up to confidential conversations. Conversing and holding the cup of tea, perhaps with two hands, acquiring warmth and confidence, Maggie's users not only experience individual pleasure of sharing, but also embrace a wider process of socialisation, generating an overall atmosphere of wellbeing. At Maggie's, the 'cup of tea' is a constant ritual involving the space and the people, the stage and the actors.

This daily ritual takes place mainly in the kitchen where the welcoming atmosphere, open space and shelves with visible and accessible utensils invite visitors to prepare their drinks and start talking, so that Maggie's stage can take on different forms of performance. In this familiar space, nothing is taken for granted: furniture, lamps, ceramics, colours and patterns are very carefully chosen to create a scenography that acts as a backdrop to the choreography of people who walk calmly or move faster during the activities. Based on this, Maggie's generates 'reflexivity', which is not only part of the daily performance but becomes real: the warm and sophisticated environment really shapes the people, who 'bend' and change around it. Indeed, through design, the performance can be charged with meaning and the subject can become an 'active agent' which, consequently, enhances the reflexivity of architecture seen as an active rather than a passive context (Hensel, 2010).

> The Maggie's centre gives you a sense of worth because you are not a patient here. In that building over there [hospital], you are a patient, but here it is you; you have your identity back.
>
> (*Focus-group Oldham*)

With reference to agency, at Maggie's the concept of the body is no longer that of the passive patient and the environment makes no difference in gender. By eliminating sex/gender distinction, Butler (1990) argues that there is no sex that is not always already gender, and that the new 'subject' is characterised by agency. Although there has never been a sex/gender distinction in the way the design of a

Maggie's centre assigns the different areas of the building, in the past, showing control and agency was different for men and women, and architecture played a role in this. The intricate structure of Maggie's Dundee's (2003) wooden ceiling reveals a hint of masculinity that solicits interest in men and balances out the emotional experience of the bright kitchen traditionally deemed to be feminine. The reasons behind the latter relate to objective facts (breast cancer was the earliest and most widespread type of cancer) and social and cultural conditions (women are more likely to open up and share). With the start of Maggie's 'men's group', the previous connotation has been, if not eliminated, at least rebalanced to a more neutral character. With no doubt, as two male participants stated, the kitchen is the place where they have the most control. In fact, in evoking atmospheres and feelings, the smell of food makes no distinctions of sex/gender. "Architecture is not about form; it is about many other things. The light and the use, and the structure, and the shadow, the smell and so on" (Zumthor, 2013, para. 2).

Movement as 'Fluid Dance'

The sense of agency and freedom of action achieved in a Maggie's centre, where open space induces movement, is further enhanced by activities such as dance, which since the ancient Greeks was a way to forget pain and worries (Raso, 2015). Considered the rediscovery of "one of the secrets of Greek education" (Sadler, 1913, quoted in Mallgrave, 2013, p. 5), at the beginning of the last century, at the Hellerau Theatre (which paved the way for the conception of the Bauhaus), Jaques-Dalcroze's "rhythmic gymnastics", also called "eurythmics", helped students be more creative and happier, making them move by listening to their body's biological rhythm (Jaques-Dalcroze, 1913, cited in Mallgrave, 2013, p. 4). Equally considered a fact "that existed in ancient times" (Laban and Ullmann 1960, p. 13), for the Hungarian dancer, choreographer and dance theorist Rudolf Laban (1879–1958) dance established the analogy between human movement and architecture. Finally, introduced in America in psychiatric facilities at the end of the Second World War, dance was revisited by Trudi Schoop and Marian Chace (Cerruto, 2018) rediscovering the idea of its therapeutic value.

At Maggie's Barts, unique in this sense among all the centres, in 2019 they used to offer the 'move–dance–feel' course, a very popular dance–therapy course for women affected by cancer (Movedancefeel, 2022). Indeed, it develops strength and positivity, and even if there are days when people are tired and don't feel like attending the course, they make great efforts to overcome the difficulties.

> One time, I came in to do the move–dance–feel class and I knew I had to do that class because, by the end of the class, my mood would improve; but while I was doing it, everyone else could see that I wasn't in my mood normally cheerful. They just gave me the space to relax and didn't force me to talk or do something I didn't want to. So, they all understood. And it's the same in any activity or space in this building. Everyone understands that cancer is not simple, you

can go forward, you can go back, you can go sideways. We all understand this, so we are all empathetic towards the situation, whatever it is. And this is the peculiarity of this building. It helps you keep your balance in this dance.

(*Move-along Barts_no. 5*)

The move–dance–feel course at Maggie's Barts, which I also attended, helped me understand that movement is what connects architecture to psychological flexibility. The dance movement performed in a favourable environment, in addition to recalling the body–mind unity of the individual, generates wellbeing by placing the internal world in continuity with the external one (Palumbo, 2011). In this phase, the mind undergoes a mutation: by releasing thoughts and tensions hitherto imprisoned in the body, the brain becomes more present and receptive, rediscovering a state of *flexibility*. By developing greater interaction with themselves and with the environment around them, people feel the presence of others and, through a chain reaction, they transmit it to everyone, in a collective ritual leading people to have a strong sense of community (Cerruto, 2018).

Movement as 'Motility'

Even if it cannot be defined in this way, movement is a displacement or a change of position.

(Merleau-Ponty, 2012 [1945], p. 279)

At Maggie's architecture invites bodily motility, that is, that property of the living organism to actively and reversibly change its position with respect to the environment and, in humans, that complex of motor manifestations considered independently of psychic activity (Treccani, 2022). For Merleau-Ponty the motility of the body in space is that series of "movements that are immediate (in the sense that they are not mediated by conscious movements, reflective, deliberative) and intentional at the same time" (Dillon, 1997, quoted by Ferri, 2006–2008, p. 94). What matters is not 'being' in space, but 'living' in space that becomes "bodily space", that is, the one in which "the object can appear as the end of our action" (Merleau-Ponty, 2012 [1945], p. 105). And this is possible only if movement, which connects the body with the world, is animated by "original intentionality" and activated by a "function of projection". Only if projected towards a goal, the movement of the subject finds meaning.

The movement of the body can perform a function in the perception of the world only if it is itself an original intentionality, a way of referring to the object distinct from knowledge. The world must be around us, not as a system of objects of which we synthesise, but as an open set of things towards which we project ourselves.

(Merleau-Ponty, 1963 [1942], cited in Ferri, 2006–2008, p. 93)

When we enter a Maggie's centre, we are immediately drawn to a view. At Maggie's Dundee, it is that of the natural landscape that opens up before us and into which we feel literally catapulted; at Maggie's Barts, it is the one of the grand luminous space to which, going up the large spiral staircase, we feel attracted; and at Maggie's Old-ham, it is the void contained in the curved glass case in which a silver birch moves that captures us and projects us towards the sky above or towards the garden below. When we try to move, the different curves of the glass case, depending on our mood, push us to the right, towards the welcome area, or to the left, towards the kitchen. In this dynamic sequence we realise that there is something that pushes us in the space, but we still don't understand what it is. As we will see in Chapter 6, it is this elusive feeling that gives rise to Maggie's therapeutic power (Figures 2.4–2.6).

Movement and 'Perception'

For architects who want to activate emotions and feelings in people, the idea of experience as a 'fusion' between the body in motion and the space that surrounds it or as a continuous interaction between perception and action is fundamental (Hale, 2017). Since action is the way in which people occupy space and through which they make themselves visible to others (Di Fazio, 2015), there can be no perception of space and others without movement. At Maggie's, the careful design strategy underlying the concept of 'spatial interaction rather than walls', which gives life to the synergy between people and place that allows a state of psychological flex-ibility, subtly pushes people to act by stimulating their perception. According to Damasio (1994), the process in a thinking organism that allows for action, is as follows:

> Having a mind means that an organism forms neural representations which can become images, be manipulated in a process called thought, and eventually in-fluence behaviour by helping predict the future, plan accordingly, and choose the next action.
>
> (Damasio 1994, p. 90)

With a holistic approach, even Berthoz in his book *The Sense of Movement* (2000) tells us that 'perception' is much more than the interpretation of messages coming from our senses; it implies simulation of action, judgement and decision–making and anticipation of the consequences of action. "The brain is above all a biological machine for moving quickly while anticipating" (2000, p. 4). Once engaged in an action, the brain formulates hypotheses on the state of some receptors and, draw-ing on memory, refers to past events to predict the consequences of the action and, combining motor and sensory signals, represents the process necessary to carry out a movement or achieve a goal. Berthoz (2000) gives the example of the skier, who cannot limit himself/herself only to continuously checking sensory signals and correcting the trajectory, but must also mentally check the race, anticipate its stages and the state of his/her sensory receptors, foresee how to correct any errors, take chances and decide before making any move. The receptors, which grouped

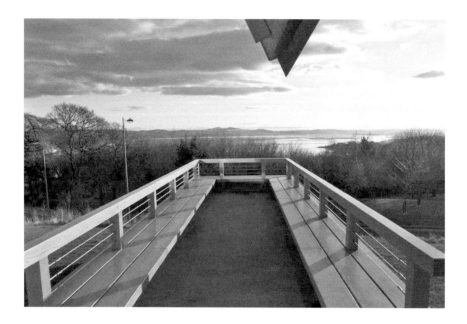

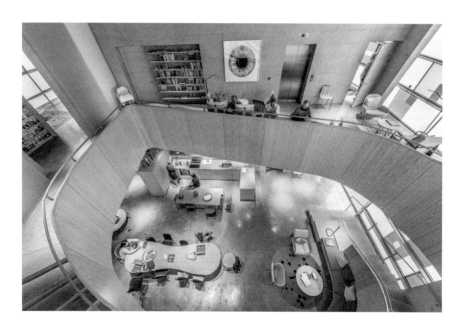

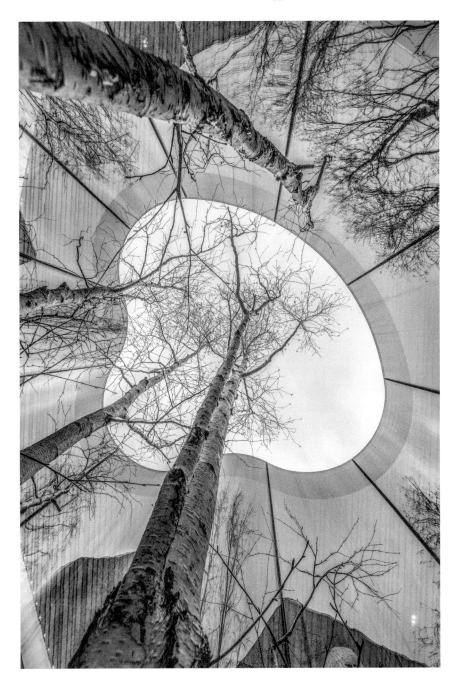

FIGURES 2.4–2.6 Maggie's Dundee (2003) (Courtesy of Maggie's), Maggie's Barts (2017) and Maggie's Oldham (2017) (©Marco Castelli Nirmal). Entering Maggie's buildings there is a sense of projection.

together are called "configurations", are collectively responsible for what is called "sense of movement" or *kinesthesia* (or 'sixth sense').

> *Kinesthesia* is the result of cooperation among several sensors, and it requires the brain to coherently reconstruct movement in the body and in the environment.
>
> (Berthoz, 2000, p. 5)

As Berthoz (2000) explains, there are more than five receptors that contribute to the sense of movement—even eight or nine if we include the muscle–proprioceptive, skin, visual and vestibular (inner ear) receptors—and the information that reaches the brain arrives in a holistic way and with different paths; it is this that gives the brain the proprioceptive role, that is, the ability to recognise the position of the body in space and the speed of contraction and stretch of the muscles, even without the support of vision. From a neuroscientific point of view, in fact, it is not true that vision always has primacy over the other senses, as it is precisely the remarkable ability of the brain that allows it to choose which sense or which combination of senses is relevant for a given movement (Berthoz, 2000). Once again, it is thanks to movement that we perceive the world.

Already at the foundation of Marleau-Ponty's theory of perception (2012 [1945]), for a scientific clarification why movement is essential to perception, we must refer to the discovery of mirror neurons that demonstrated the link between perception and action.

In the 1980s, a group of scientists from Parma (Italy) led by Giacomo Rizzolatti and composed of Luciano Fadiga, Leonardo Fogassi, Vittorio Gallese and Giuseppe di Pellegrino, who was engaged in the study of the premotor cortex of the monkey (area F5), had accidentally discovered that those neurons—later called "mirror neurons" because they 'mirror' the action of others—which discharged when a monkey performed an action (for example, grasping a banana and bringing it to its mouth), also 'fired' when it observed "specific, meaningful hand movements performed by the experimenters" (di Pellegrino et al., 1992, p.1). From a physiological point of view, the novelty of this discovery and following investigations came from the fact that motor neurons, gave 'visual' responses.

> Perhaps one of the most interesting aspects of this discovery consists in the fact that, for the first time, a neural mechanism has been identified which allows a direct translation between the sensory (visual and auditory) description of a motor act and its execution. This coupling system allows you to translate the results of the visual analysis of an observed movement into something that the observer is able to understand, to the extent that the observer already possesses it pragmatically and experientially.
>
> (Gallese, 2009, p. 9*)

In addition to the visual-motor correlation, this discovery had highlighted how, at the basis of the activation of these neurons, generated by an action, there is

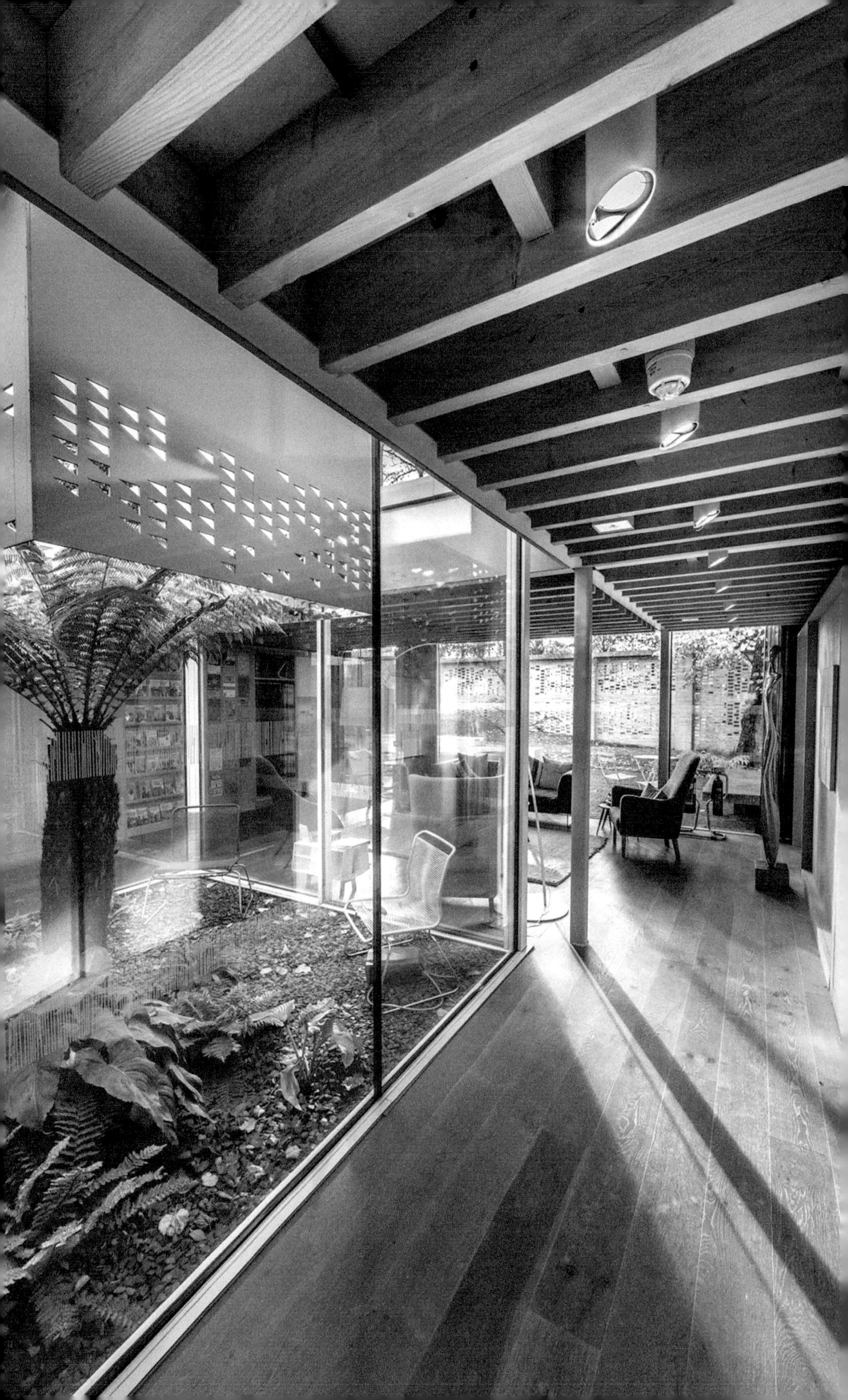

always the purpose of that action (in this case, eating the banana). In other words, an object always has an intentional value and a purpose. "Seeing the object means automatically evoke what we would do with that object" (Gallese, 2006, p. 301*). This means that objects are not only identified, differentiated and categorised by the brain by virtue of their physical 'appearance', but also in relation to the effects of interaction with an agent. "It is therefore exclusively the agent-object relationship that evokes the activation of mirror-neurons" (Gallese 2006, p. 305*).

In the 1990s, the team succeed to demonstrating that mirror neurons also exist in humans, proving that human action—i.e. a motor act aimed at achieving a goal—is the consequence of a visible, understandable and therefore imitable intention as there is a "process of motor equivalence between what is acted out and what is perceived" (Gallese, 2006, p. 304*). With this discovery, which no longer looked at the relationship with the object but at the social dimension of the 'organism–world' relationship, it became clear that *mirroring* allows us to experience the motor actions of others (even without moving our bodies) and to understand the meanings of their intentions, pushing us to equate what others do with what we can do as observers, in a "non—conscious, automatic and pre-linguistic mechanism of motor simulation" (Gallese, 2006, p. 304*). Providing a scientific explanation for the imitation and sharing of intentions already outlined by Merleau-Ponty (2012 [1945]) and establishing a fundamental precedent of the fact that our brain is able to simulate the action of others through perception, Rizzolatti's discovery demonstrated at a neuronal level, for the first time, the link between perception and action, confirming that the motor system and the perceptual system work together, in unison: by capturing the intentionality of the other, we reproduce the 'movement' and simulate it within ourselves (Gallese, 2006 cited by Di Fazio, 2015). In conclusion, "perceiving an action—and understanding its meaning—is equivalent to simulating it internally" (Gallese, 2006, p. 304*).

In neuroscience, this link had already been hypothesised by many before Rizzolatti, in a series of studies that go under the name of 'Simulation Theory'. As Berthoz explains, borrowing from Janet (1935, cited in Berthoz, 2000, p. 10), an example of simulated action is when we see an armchair and perceive its comfort before sitting on it: we already have within us the action that we associate with the armchair, which we call 'perceptual pattern', and which Merleau-Ponty described well: "Vision is the brain's way of touching" (Merleau-Ponty, 1964, quoted in Berthoz, 2000, p. 11). In spatial perception, these 'perceptual patterns' direct our emotions, behaviours and memories through neuronal activation patterns to which each perceptual pattern is associated, "a repertoire of pre-perceptions connected to a repertoire of actions" (Berthoz, 2000, p. 20). In the perceptual process, the predictive power of the brain increases because the brain processes information holistically (Damasio, 1989 cited by Berthoz, 2000). However, there is no perception of space unless associated with an emotion and no emotion can arise if it is not linked to movement.

> There is no perception of space or movement, no vertigo or loss of balance, no caress given or received, no sound heard or uttered, no gesture of capture or

grasping that is not accompanied by emotion or induced by it. But it is necessary to construct a physiology of relationships between movement and emotion.

(Berthoz, 2000, p. 7)

Hybrid

Although not much considered by Maggie's co-clients at the time of our interview, the hybrid has always been central to Charles Jencks' since 1985. Respecting the wishes of his wife Maggie who had a "long list of everything" to put into the small building, a single 'whole', Charles has always been convinced that this multiple and heterogeneous nature gave the building a 'power' that enhances architectural richness and human values. The hybrid nature of the Maggie's centre is revealed, above all, in its undefined space, made up of a series of spaces that follow one another and overlap, which become, when necessary, the non-home house, the non-institutional collective hospital, the non-religious church, the non-museum art gallery. Ambiguous and transformative, Maggie's hybrid proved to be the second element characterising the therapeutic environment of the Maggie's centre.

Hybrid as 'Ambiguity' and 'Mutability'

In the scientific and social disciplines (biology, sociology, anthropology), from Mendel (1822–1884) onwards, the meaning of hybrid has almost always been negative, because it was linked to the idea of a "crossing or mixing"–often with a monstrous connotation–of beings that are hardly compatible with each other (Cambridge Dictionary, 2023a). In architecture, however, the combination of multiple functions within a single structure has always been a valid strategy that has been repeated throughout history: the building above the bridge, the apartment above the shop, the Roman baths which included many functions (Avitabile, 2013). Unlike multifunctional buildings (e.g., shopping centres), where multiple functions simply coexist, hybrid buildings implement an interaction between functions that are necessary for each other's life, cultivating a 'reciprocal alliance' (Fenton, 1985). In this coexistence, there is no hierarchy and ambiguity is seen as a virtue.

The term 'ambiguity', from the Latin *ambigĕre* (=to push one thing from two sides), indicates a lack of clarity (Cambridge Dictionary, 2023b), which in art is an intrinsic characteristic of the aesthetic representation itself. As Calanca (1991) reminds us, in the *Poetics* (334–330 B.C., Chapter 1) Aristotle tells us that all art is mimetic and makes use of other arts either separately or in combination, and does not release aesthetic information unless associated with unknown and unexpected elements. Ambiguity, therefore, is identified with the very concept of art and, as such, becomes not only its characteristic, but also a source of delight.

In the "non-type building", as Jencks defined the Maggie's centre (2015, p. 28), the four faces of the hybrid intervene simultaneously or one at a time, manifesting themselves more or less evidently depending on the individual, transforming and adapting to people's feelings. This ability of the hybrid to change, or rather its characteristic of presenting itself in different forms even in an unpredictable way, is called 'mutability'. In the case of the processes of mutation and metamorphosis, since ancient times, reference has been made to a dynamic conception of form. To better illustrate this concept, Calanca (1991) refers to Arnheim when, in his book *The Dynamics of the Architectural Form* (1977), he compares the device used by the architect in creating a building that generates mutability and transition to that used by Richard Wagner in his music to generate the phenomenon of "enharmonic modulation" described as follows:

> (...) the almost imperceptible shift from one key to another, in the course of which certain tones act as bridges by fulfilling different functions in the two keys and thereby display a double allegiance. The transitional moment generates a slight sensation of seasickness, unwelcome or exhilarating depending on the listener's disposition, because the frame of reference is temporarily lost.
>
> (Arnheim, 1977, p. 167)

Arnheim defines this device (including the transitional phase of disorientation) as an effective stylistic means of expressing liberation from absolute standards (Calanca, 1991). Lived as a 'sonata', the spatial experience in architecture is a perceptual sequence that presents pauses and sudden changes. After a moment of bewilderment, due to the indefinite, changing, compelling space, Maggie's visitors find their balance in the new context. Although initially it can create disorientation, the multiple space of the hybrid induces, in the following moment, a feeling of wellbeing and the beginning of a new experience.

> Sometimes, it's kind of scary when you come in, I never saw a building like this before. But, after a while, you feel proud of it, it is so special.
>
> (*Focus-group Barts*)

Reaffirming 'ambiguity' and 'mutability' as characteristics of Maggie's hybrid means, ultimately, underlining the holistic and all-encompassing nature of the Maggie's centre, confirming once and for all the hybrid power claimed by Charles Jencks (1985). As he argued, the hybrid is complex and contradictory, because it must have open and closed spaces, be welcoming and informal like a home, but clear and discreet in order not to impose itself, yet, at times, even provocative. This skillful interweaving of open and semi-open spaces has the important function of maintaining direct contact with the visitors (Jencks, 2018) and help Maggie's staff keep control of everything that happens in the building. In fact, the concept of 'hybrid' is also appropriate for people who, coming from different worlds and with multiple tasks assigned, have many skills. When they were nurses, staff members could not fill other roles, also because the layout of their workspace did not allow it. At Maggie's, supported by the building in many ways, the staff manages to carry out many of them, including the fundamental one of offering 'a cup of tea'.

Hybrids that Evolve

In healthcare, the ever-evolving Maggie's centre, never completed and which has already spawned 30 or more centres, shows the potential to become a model and,

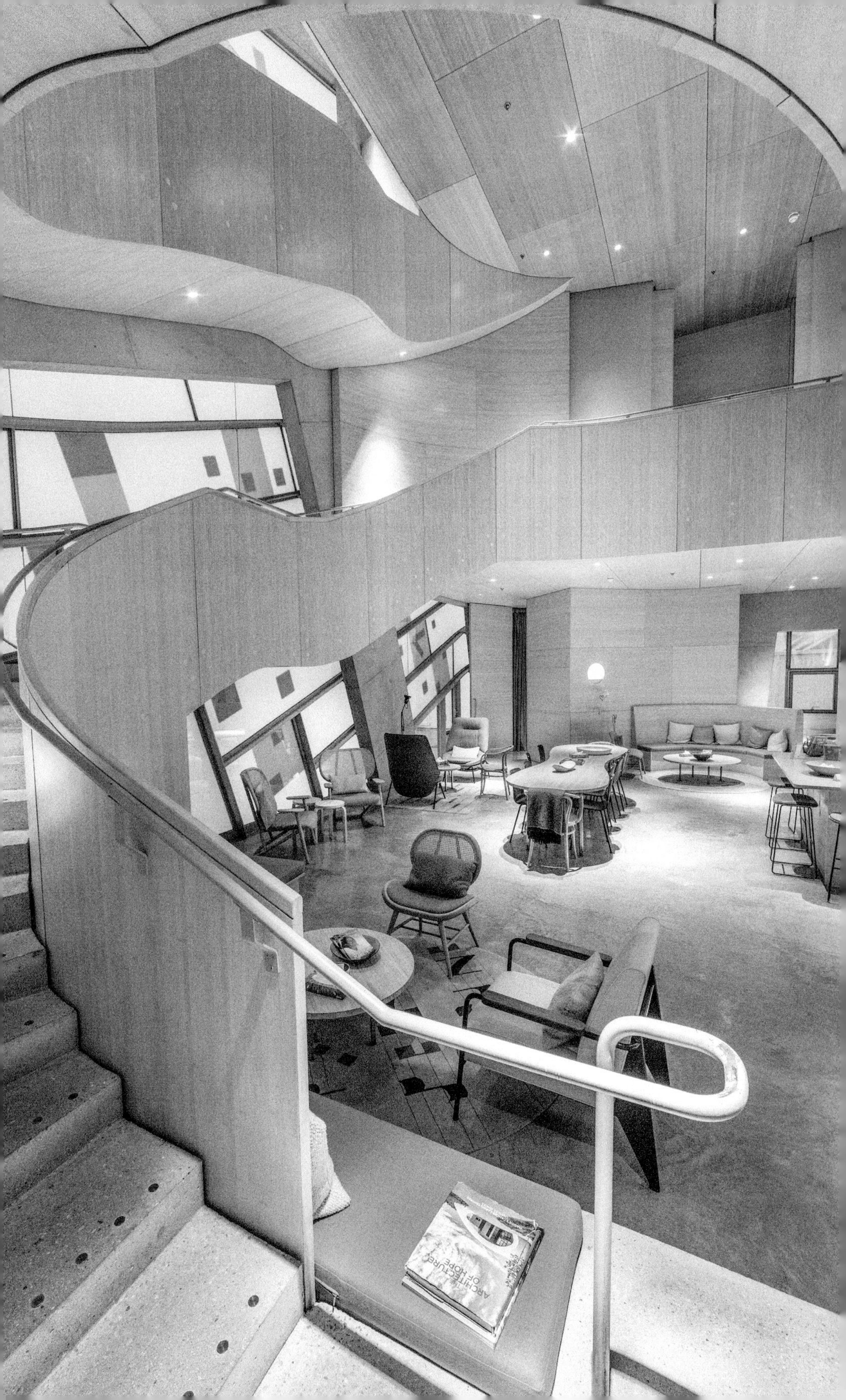
ARCHITECTURE
OF HOPE

thanks to its multifaceted and heterogeneous nature which gives its buildings a power—a hybrid one—perhaps a paradigm. To make a contribution to the 'Construction of Health', as a model or, rather, as a paradigm, as we will see in Chapter 7, I will here explore historical hybrids that have evolved, first investigating the concept of the evolution of the model.

The concept of evolution of a model in architecture can be compared, in music, to the 'variation on a theme' dating back to ancient Greece. In this process, the original melody is transformed into a succession of variations, in which each variation, while remaining recognisable, becomes a new piece in itself. In the evolution of the plan of Frank Gehry's design for the Peter Lewis House—for which Maggie Keswick designed the garden—as the narrator of the film "A Constructive Madness" (Dailymotion, 2002) explains, the way it varies is similar to that of J.S. Bach's Goldberg Variations (1741). At the beginning of the music, the basic theme is almost inaudible; however, over the next 30 pieces of music, this theme varies so much to the point that it gives birth to new music of such ingenious invention that the listener is completely distracted from what is happening in the composer's basic plan. As with the Goldberg Variations, each of Gehry's planimetric variations is distinct, indeed, "an autonomous expression of a different universal fusion". In the book *Variations of Identity. Type in Architecture*, considering variation as a typological procedure, Carlos Martí Aris (2021) legitimises the transformation and development of a given theme as a fundamental principle of configuration. Without repetition it is difficult to speak of type, but repetition cannot be generated without difference.

The concept of evolution includes, in fact, that of difference, due, however, not so much to the speculation of multiple design solutions as in the case of Gerhry, but rather to a spontaneous phenomenon of adaptation to the different geographical, cultural, social conditions of the place or stylistic trends of the time. In antiquity this type of adaptation process was typical of hybrid complexes such as the already seen healing temples dedicated to the god Asclepius (V B.C.–IV A.D.), which multiplied by the hundreds over the vast Hellenic territory, repeating the same architectural components (*Asclepeion, abaton, katagòghion*, theatre, etc.), but changing layout to adapt to different sites. The same goes for the Benedictine Monastery (530 A.D.), which thanks to its hybrid character of religious, charitable, artistic, agricultural contents, had been reproduced by the thousands throughout Europe with different subcategories (such as abbeys and convents), maintaining the same components (church, library, oratory, refectory, etc.), taking on different forms to adapt to the new site. As Yago Bonet Correa states "every place is sacred because it is unique in relation to the universe" (2000, p. 53*); therefore, when architecture undertakes the construction of a place, it deduces its specificities from it. For example, within the evolution of the monastic complex, the more recent Monastery of La Tourette by Le Corbusier (1960), while remaining faithful to the traditional form of enclosure inspired by the Certosa di Galluzzo (Florence), seeks a link with the external natural context, elevating and offering the monks glimpses of suggestive land-scapes. Furthermore, by accepting the meaning and form of the cloister, work-ing in plan and section, Le Corbusier reinterprets its traditional circulatory and social functions around and within the cloister to create a system of movement, which becomes the organising principle of the monastery (Lloyd, 1989). From the Latin *claustrum* (=separated from the world), the cloister constitutes the heart of the monastery, the internal 'void', source of light and air, meeting point for the monks for prayer and social life, but also its matrix which, even in the modern version, has never changed (Zucchi, 1989). In the evolution of the ty-pology, the constant element around which the building complex transforms, is what, as we shall see in Chapter 7, gives the type the strength to become a model or paradigm.

Non-Therapeutic/Therapeutic

If we think of the healing architecture of Greek temples, Maggie's centres con-tain all the ingredients of the *therapeutikós* space: the splendid architecture, the glimpses of nature, the presence of professionals who provide care in synergy with the building, the multiple functions, the openness to family members, the 'mind-as-important-as-the-body' message. Despite this, the Maggie's centre shows no signs of the therapeutic environment typical of modern healthcare, quite the op-posite: non-clinical, small in size, with a quiet, pleasant, reassuring atmosphere. In this, it helps that the organisation has dropped the suffix 'Cancer Care', and more recently that of 'Centre'. Consequently, when they say they go to "Mag-gie's", visitors are often misunderstood, and those who are not familiar with the place might think they refer to a disco or a gym. Yet, rather strangely, as we saw with the hybrid, ambiguity helps people to feel normal, which, for a person with cancer, means feeling good. This technique of 'low definition' is also adopted in the dissemination of the support programme with a limited use of written words. For example, the brochure that simply says 'Just come in' is a way to get people into the centre where they will receive information by voice, directly from the staff. In particular, the absence of the term 'therapeutic' in the staff language helps divert attention from the cancer. Paradoxically, not using the term therapeutic generates a therapeutic effect.

Absence of Signs of Sanitary Architecture

As we saw in the introduction, the goal of neuroscience is to explain what Merleau-Ponty had already predicted a long time ago, namely how the body and the mind are one and work together in the perception of reality. However, when an illness occurs, the perception we have of our body as an embodiment of the mind changes. Recognising a weakness of the flesh in relation to the mind (and conscience), the sick go back to seeing their body as an aggregate of organs which, referring to the old division between body and soul, separets from their consciousness (Merleau-Ponty, 2012 [1945], cited in Di Fazio, 2015). In a hospital, this condition places the patient in an inferior condition. As Foucault argued in his *The Birth of the Clinic* (1973 [1963]), the 'clinic', as it has been conceived since the end of the eighteenth century, is based on the relationship with the patient's body, but not with his/her person. Contrary to this, in a Maggie's centre, the architecture devoid of sanitary signs is what initiates the process of change, according to which people with cancer are invited to feel no longer as patients but as 'normal' people. In fact, the first thing visitors notice at Maggie's is the absence of the typical elements of sanitary architecture to the point that the curious passing-by enter the building attracted by the kitchen, often visible from the outside, thinking it is a restaurant or a cafe. In addition to the absence of corridors, bathrooms in a row, reception counters, alarms, badges and uniforms, the absence of signage of any kind makes the Maggie's centre feel like a home. Finally, not categorising the organisation as a healing environment and not associating particular therapeutic qualities with the environment—rightly invoked by Laura Lee on the basis that there is no scientific evidence that the Maggie's centre is a therapeutic environment—is part of well-calibrated tactics implemented by simply not placing "expectations on how people entering the door should feel" (*Lee, 18.05.2019*). Ultimately, 'absence' rather than 'presence' is the catalyst that starts the process of change, leading people to accept a new condition of life.

'The Enigma of the Obvious'

As the title borrowed from Armezzani (2019) implies, the nature of the Maggie's centre is enigmatic and contradictory. For Laura Lee, one of the things that the architecture at Maggie's has been able to offer is, in fact, to provide the opposite things that cancer patients often talk about in the hospital environment, where they feel helpless and hopeless, alone and isolated, out of control. The Maggie's centre is designed to make people feel responsible by telling them that "this is their place", a unique way to help people connect with each other (*Lee, 16.10.2019*).

When people with cancer cross the threshold, they are free to decide whether or not to accept help from the staff and without having to register, visitors can behave as if they were at home. Within a space that instils safety and control, visitors can navigate the process of change at their own pace. Thanks to the way the building is designed and the continuous open spaces, people with cancer can wander, observe, simulate others and react. Given its hybrid nature, everyone is free to consider the Maggie's centre as they wish: a home away from home, a spiritual place, a place to receive psychological, practical or lifestyle support, a pleasant place to meet new friends and laugh or cry with them. By doing the opposite of the obvious, i.e. giving people freedom of choice, Maggie's strategically gains the trust of people who become willing to open up and share experiences and emotions.

As mentioned, to satisfy all the activities foreseen in the timetable, during the day the staff constantly moves the furnishings and the rooms continuously change their setting to become a new space every time. The flexibility of the physical space also lies in the fact that the building has no secrets, and nothing hides behind the doors which, instead of closing, slide or rotate because, in this way, they can always "be left a little open". Thanks to the way the building is designed, many confidential conversations can take place comfortably in the same room and people feel reassured that what they say will stay inside the building. By doing the opposite of the obvious, i.e. offering flexibility and versatility, Maggie's buildings strategically transfer control to people who, by adapting easily, will become more flexible.

At the base of everything, however, is the invitation to normality, that is, to no longer feel like a hospital patient, but a normal person. When people with cancer enter the hospital, they feel and behave like patients; as a result, the family treats their loved ones as vulnerable or as someone who is no longer 'normal'. When they arrive at Maggie's, people stop acting like patients and suddenly feel normal again and this happens because both the staff and the building remind them of who they are. This practice of 'normalisation' is evident in several aspects of Maggie's programme: from sitting alone and reading a book just like at home, to sharing heartwarming stories around the kitchen table, to participating in physical activities that for people with cancer are sometimes challenging but empowering. By doing the opposite of the obvious, i.e. treating people not as sick but encouraging them to behave normally in a normal environment, Maggie strategically gains people's reaction and the healing process to begin.

The technique of the opposite of the obvious can be found in psychology under the name of 'Reverse Psychology'. This practice is used to get people to do or say something by telling them the opposite of what you want them to achieve. In today's healthcare, freedom, flexibility, and normality certainly do not characterise a therapeutic environment; on the contrary, in a Maggie's centre, all these aspects are what allow visitors to experience the beneficial effects typical of a therapeutic environment. Whether intentionally or not, with her intuition of declaring that the Maggie's centre is not a therapeutic environment, leaving openness and freedom to any interpretation, Laura Lee applies one of the most effective persuasion techniques and cognitive modalities. In phenomenology, intuition is considered a methodology of knowledge that implies openness, questioning, and taking nothing for granted. In fact, "one cannot speak of an objective reality and a false one, it is simply a question of comparing two points of view, two perspectives" (Armezzani, 2019, p. 6*). This methodology has no certainties and knowledge must always be questioned and renewed.

> In a sense, because we are not trying to theorise and to put assumptions on how the person coming into the door must feel, it means there is freedom in our Brief and how we work with the architect to allow for the person to find their own way. In a way, it is a bit like our programme gives support, is about the best way

for them, because everybody has a different set of stuff going on. For some people seeing the sky might be too overwhelming or too much sky.

(*Lee 18.05.2019*)

And not only does Laura Lee have the attitude that says "one cannot speak of an objective reality and a false one" denoting a phenomenological approach, but also the Maggie's centre takes nothing for granted. The phenomena that occur in a Maggie's centre are based on evidence: they are not facts that arise, but facts that are experienced and always subjectively so. As Armezzani says "if we substitute the criterion of evidence for objectivity, it can be accepted as an essential necessity that everything looks different for different subjects" (2019, p. 6*). Under this assumption, the obvious cannot be taken for granted and even what is obvious is actually enigmatic. This way of looking at the world undermines what is familiar to us, but in the long run it will be able to transform the universal evidence "into something transparent and understandable" (Armezzani, 2019 p. 7*).

How *Flexibility* Enables the Therapeutic Environment

This chapter has revealed the three elements inherent in the therapeutic environment of the Maggie's centre. In my doctoral research, after having discovered them, examined them individually and defined them as essential components of the spatial experience to produce therapeutic effects in Maggie's users, the conclusion was that it is the coexistence of the three elements that gives rise to Maggie's therapeutic environment. Inherent in all three, brought together in a single concept, this coexistence is called *flexibility*, which is what "universally" defines a therapeutic environment. At Maggie's, the dynamic spatial experience, positive and placed in a holistic context devoid of signs of sanitary architecture, generates a synergy between people and place, a 'fluid dance' that allows psychological flexibility to give rise to an engaging environment that we could define therapeutic. Since, as Viktor Frankl (2008) states, we cannot control what happens in our life, we just have to control our mind and how we respond to it, what connects us to this environment is the *flexibility* of our mental condition.

Flexibility can be illustrated, as for the Greeks, as a 'fluid dance', in which people's minds flex like reeds moved by the wind. In architecture, this feeling of mental flexibility is described with the concept of 'aura'. The *Aura*, a nymph from Greek mythology that means "breeze of wind", transmits the impact of a person, thing, or place from a distance (Theoi, 2023). As described by Walter Benjamin in his essay *The Work of Art in the Age of Mechanical Reproduction* (1935), 'aura' or "uniqueness of an object of art" is "its presence in time and space (…) the unique phenomenon of a distance, however close it may be" (Benjamin, 1935, pp. 3, 5). As an intrinsic movement of its architectural space, Maggie's *flexibility* bends people's minds, encouraging them to accept something that was previously intolerable.

If, as Alvaro Siza states (quoted in Berger and Gepshtein, 2020, 8:40), "architecture without people becomes sculpture" and, therefore, architecture is not such unless in the presence of people and if, as Howells says (2016), it is the synergy between people and place that enables psychological flexibility and makes people flexible, it is only with the presence of people that a building, an environment or a place can be therapeutic. Understood as a psychological state, being therapeutic or non-therapeutic is not a condition of the space, but, rather a subjective condition: 'therapeutic' is the *flexibility* of our mental condition. The experience of a therapeutic environment inscribes and persists in people in various ways. To generate this experience, paradoxically, Maggie's uses psychological devices such as 'absence' rather than 'presence'. Once we learn how to read its characteristics, its enigmas and contradictions, we will begin to recognise a therapeutic environment.

References

Armezzani, M. (2019) *L'enigma dell'ovvio. La fenomenologia di Husserl come fondamento di un'altra psicologia*. Università degli Studi di Padova. https://www.docsity.com/it/l-enigma-dell-ovvio-la-fenomenologia-di-husserl-come-fondamento-di-un-altra-psicologia-maria-armezzani/5018698/

Arnheim, R. (1977) *The Dynamics of Architectural Form*. Berkeley, Los Angeles, and London: University of California Press

Avitabile, F. (2013) *Prospettive ibride negli spazi urbani contemporanei*, Doctoral Thesis, Urban Design and Planning, 'Federico II' University of Naples. http://www.fedoa.unina.it/9313/1/TESI%20AVITABILE.pdf

Benjamin, W. (1935) 'The Work of Art in the Age of Mechanical Reproduction', in Arendt, H. (ed.) (1969) *Illuminations*. New York: Schocken Books, pp. 1–26

Berthoz, A. (2000) *The Brain's Sense of Movement*. Boston MA: Harvard University Press

Bonet Correa, Y. (2000) 'Construcción e natureza ou a arquitectura como a transformación positiva', *Obradoiro: revista de arquitectura y urbanismo*, 28, pp. 52–53

Butler, J. (1990) *Gender Trouble: Feminism and the Subversion of Identity*. London and New York: Routledge

Butler, J. (1993) *Bodies that Matter: On the Discursive Limits of 'Sex'*. London and New York: Routledge

Butterfield, A. and Martin, D. (2014) 'The Silent Carers: Exploring the Role of Architecture and Gardens at the Maggie's Cancer Care Centres'. *Psycho-Oncology*, 23, 318–319

Butterfield, A. and Martin, D. (2016) 'Affective Sanctuaries: Understanding Maggie's As Therapeutic Landscapes', *Landscape Research*, 41(6), pp. 695–706

Calanca, C. (1991) *L'identità ibrida: modalità dell'architettura nei paesaggi contemporanei*, Doctoral Thesis, Faculty of Architecture, Polytechnic of Milan. https://opac.biblio.polimi.it/sebina/repository/link/oggetti_digitali/fullfiles/PERL-TDDE/TESI_2004-161.PDF

Cambridge Dictionary (2023a) *Definition of Hybrid*. https://dictionary.cambridge.org/dictionary/english/hybrid

Cambridge Dictionary (2023b) *Definition of Ambiguity*. https://dictionary.cambridge.org/dictionary/english/ambiguity

Cerruto, E. (2018) *Metodologia e pratica della Danza Terapeutica*. Milan: Franco Angeli

Dailymotion (2002) A Constructive Madness. https://www.dailymotion.com/video/x2nw9m6

Damasio, A. (1994) *Descartes' Error: Emotion, Reason, and the Human Brain*. London: Vintage

Di Fazio, C. (2015) 'The Free Body. Notes on Maurice Merleau-Ponty's Phenomenology of Movement', *SIF-Praha.Cz*. https://www.sif-praha.cz/wp-content/uploads/2013/04/The-free-body.pdf

Di Pellegrino, G., Fadiga, L., Fogassi, L., Gallese, V. and Rizzolatti, G. (1992) 'Understanding Motor Events: A Neurophysiological Study', *Experimental Brain Research*, 91, pp. 176–180

Fenton, J. (1985) 'Hybrid Buildings', *Pamphlet Architecture*, 11, pp. 3–43

Ferri, G. (2006–2008) *Il Problema dell'intenzionalita' nella filosofia di Merleau-Ponty*, Doctoral Thesis, Faculty of Philosophy, University of Verona. https://iris.univr.it/handle/11562/337344

Folador, M. (2006) *L'organizzazione perfetta. La regola di San Benedetto. Una saggezza antica al servizio dell'impresa moderna*. Milan: Guerini e Associati

Foucault, M. (1973 [1963]) *The Birth of the Clinic: An Archaeology of Medical Perception*. London and New York: Routledge

Frankl, V. (2008) *Man's Search For Meaning*. London, Sidney, Auckland, Johannesburg: Rider

Frisone, C. (2021) *The Role of Architecture in the Therapeutic Environment. The Case of the Maggie's Cancer Care Centre*, Doctoral Thesis, Faculty of Technology, Design and Environment, Oxford Brookes University. https://doi.org/10.24384/0ejy-7815

Gallese, V. (2006) 'Corpo vivo, simulazione incarnata e intersoggettività: Una prospettiva neurofenomenologica', in Cappuccio, M. (ed.) *Neurofenomenologia Le Scienze della Mente*. Milan: Mondadori, pp. 293–326

Gallese, V. (2009). 'Neuroscienze e fenomenologia', Treccani Terzo Millennio, I, 1–32 https://www.treccani.it/enciclopedia/neuroscienze-e-fenomenologia_%28XXI-Secolo%29/

Hale, J. (2017) *Merleau-Ponty for Architects*. London and New York: Routledge

Hayes, S. C. and Smith, S. (2005) *Get Out of Your Mind and Into Your Life. The New Acceptance & Commitment Therapy*. Oakland, CA: New Harbinger Publications

Hensel, M. (2010) 'Performance-oriented Architecture', *FORMakademisk*, 3(1), pp. 36–56

Howells, L. (2016) *Synergy between People and Place*, 8 June. https://www.youtube.com/watch?v=tvE78D30CbQ

Jencks, C. (1985) *Modern Movements in Architecture*. London: Penguin Group

Jencks, C. (2015) *The Architecture of Hope: Maggie's Cancer Caring Centres* (2nd ed.). London: Frances Lincoln

Kearney, M. (2009) *A Place of Healing: Working with Nature & Soul at the End of Life*. New Orleans: Spring Journal Books

Kusenbach, M. (2003) 'Street Phenomenology: The Go-along As Ethnographic Research Tool', *Ethnography*, 4, pp. 455–485

Laban, R. and Ullmann, L. (1960) *The Mastery of movement*. London: Mac Donald and Evans

Latham, A. (2003) 'Research, Performance and Doing Human Geography: Some Reflections on the Diary-Photograph, Diary-Interview Method', *Environment and Planning A: Economy and Space*, 35, pp. 1993–2017

Lloyd, P. (1989) *A Convention Center: A Typological Approach to the Design of an Institutional Building*, M.Arch Thesis, MIT https://citeseerx.ist.psu.edu/document?repid=rep1&type=pdf&doi=0e67e2fcfe885cda50ac52ecd19ff86ca8dbdb50

Mallgrave, H.F. (2013) *Architecture and Embodiment. The Implications of the New Sciences and Humanities for Design*. London and New York: Routledge

Martí Arís, C. (2021) *Variation of Identity - Type in Architecture* (transl. by Claudia Mion and Fabio Licitra) Dijon: Les Presses du Réel

Martin, D. (2014). 'The Choreography of The Kitchen Table: The Agency of Everyday Spaces in the Experience of Care'. *Psycho-Oncology*, 23, 203–204.

Martin, D. (2016) 'Curating Space, Choreographing Care: The Efficacy of The Everyday', in Bates, C., Imrie, R. and Kullman, K. (eds.) *Care and Design: Bodies, Buildings, Cities*. Oxford: Wiley, pp. 39–57

Martin, D. (2017) 'Between Bodies and Buildings: The Place of Comfort within Therapeutic Spaces', in Crang, P., McNally, D. and Price, L. (eds.) *Geographies of Comfort*. London: Ashgate/Routledge

Martin, D., Nettleton, S. and Buse C. (2019) 'Affecting Care: Maggie's Centres and the Orchestration of Architectural Atmospheres', *Social Science & Medicine*, 240, pp. 1–8

Merleau-Ponty, M. (1963 [1942]) *The Structure of Behaviour*. Translated by A. L. Fisher. Boston, MA: Beacon

Merleau-Ponty, M. (2012 [1945]) *Phenomenology of Perception*. Translated by D. A. Landes. Abington and New York: Routledge

Movedancefeel (2022) Move Dance Feel. https://www.movedancefeel.com/

Palumbo, C. (2011) *La Danza-Educativa: Dimensioni Formative E Prospettive Educative*. Vol. 1. Doctoral Thesis, Dipartimento Di Scienze Umane, Filosofiche E Della Formazione, Università Degli Studi Di Salerno

Raso, M. (2015) 'La danza nell'antica Grecia, un esempio culturale da imitare', *DanzaNews. it*, 15 June. http://www.danzanews.it/la-danza-nellantica-grecia-un-esempio-culturale-da-imitare/

Rose, G., Degen, M. and Basdas, B. (2010) 'More on Big Things: Building Events and Feelings', *Transactions of the Institute of British Geographers*, 35, pp. 334–349

Theoi (2023) 'Definition of Aura'. https://www.theoi.com/Nymphe/Aurai.html

Treccani (2022) 'Definition of Motility'. https://www.treccani.it/vocabolario/motilita/

Zucchi, C. (1989) *L'Architettura dei cortili milanesi. 1535–1706*. Milan: Electa

Zumthor, P. (2013) 'Architecture Is Not About Form'. Interview with Peter Zumthor. Interviewed by A. Frearson for Dezeen, 6 February. https://www.dezeen.com/2013/02/06/peter-zumthor-at-the-royal-gold-medal-lecture-2013/

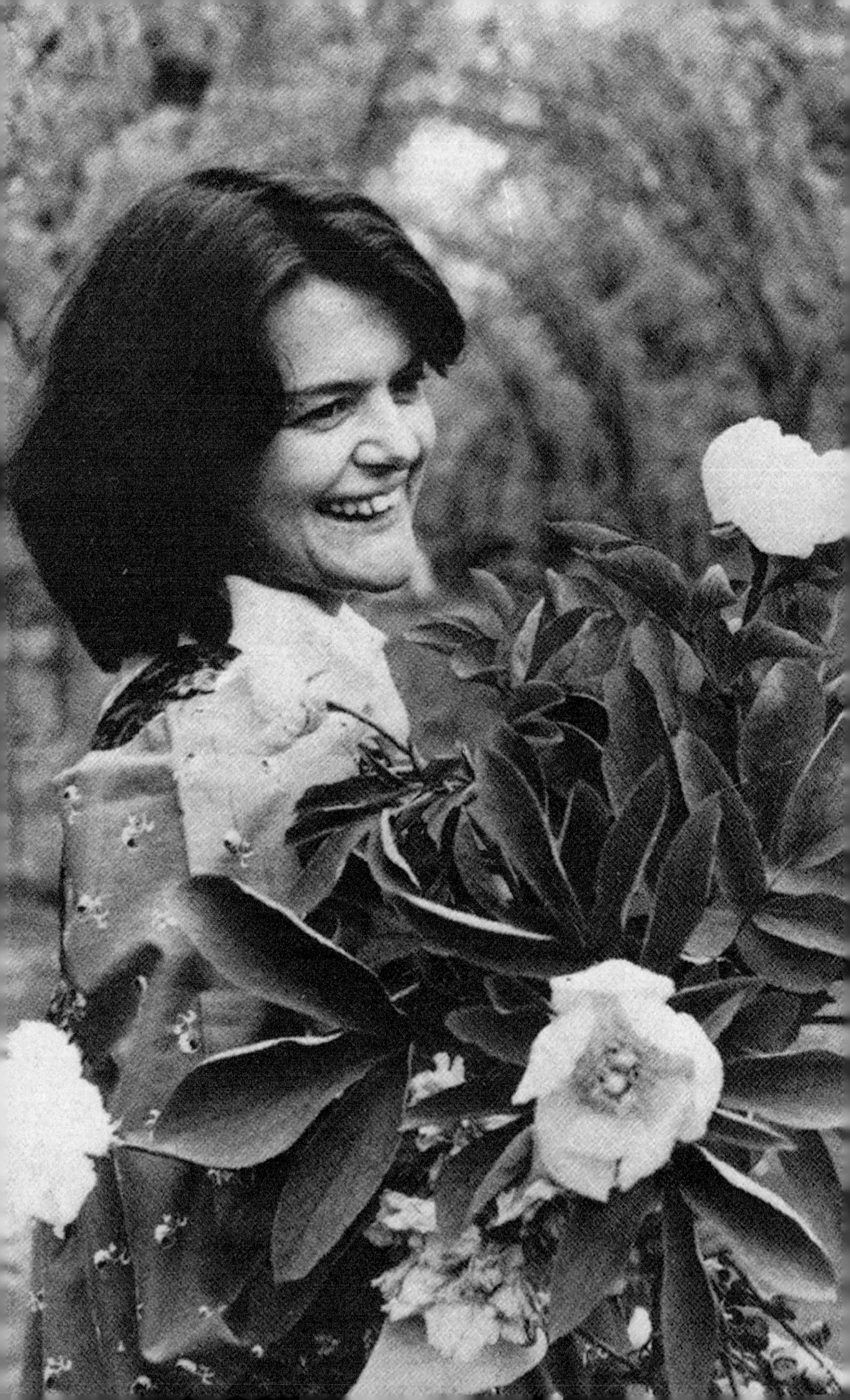

3

THE MAGGIE'S CENTRE

Maggie Keswick: Origins and Developments of the Maggie's Centre

Maggie Keswick (1941–1995) was a fashion designer with a special interest in Chinese gardens. This stemmed from her youthful experience when she, the daughter of a Scottish merchant, often travelled to China with her family, making her develop a sensitive personality and a deep passion for oriental culture. In her book *The Chinese Garden: History, Art and Architecture* (1978), Maggie had highlighted the idea that, by miniaturising the landscape, human beings can reach a more immediate harmony with nature. The book was published in 1978, the same year she married Charles Jencks (1939–2019), an American-trained architect who was young, and had therefore developed counter-current architectural theories influencing architects, theorists and critics of postmodern architecture.

Maggie and Charles had met in London in the early 1970s, when he was a lecturer and she was a student at the AA (Architectural Association). Together they travelled everywhere, even with their two children Lily and John. They visited Europe and, among the many places they visited, the *Hospices de Beaune* in France and the *Epidaurus* healing complex in Greece strongly influenced their minds to the point that, many years later, they re-emerged in the Maggie's centre. Given their shared passion for landscape architecture, Maggie and Charles worked together and, for Maggie's family, transformed the 30-acre garden of the Portrack House in Dumfriesshire, Scotland, into the 'Garden of Cosmic Speculation'. In it, Jencks designed the Garden of the Six Senses, in which he placed the metal installation representing Maggie peering into a brain through her fingers, a celebration of her sixth sense which Maggie, when alive, manifested with "finger-waggling".

DOI: 10.4324/9781003244516-3

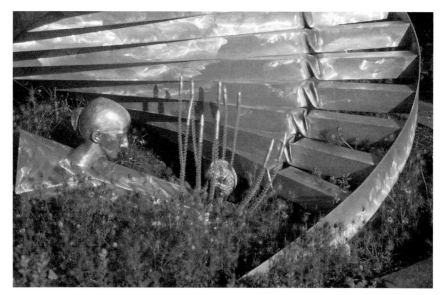

FIGURE 3.1   Charles Jencks' metal installation depicting Maggie peering into her brain in the Garden of the Six Senses at Maggie's family's Portrack House in Dumfriesshire, Scotland (Courtesy of Charles Jencks).

> The sixth sense is the female sense of anticipation as a metaphorical sense, a sense in the end of the fingertips, of the mood and direction to go. Intuition.
>
> *(Jencks, 18.06.2018)*

Just like Willis' *Cerebri Anatome* seen in the introduction, the image of this installation also seems very representative of the purpose of this book (Figure 3.1).

Even separately, Charles and Maggie had extraordinary lives. When they were in Los Angeles in the 1980s, while Charles was lecturing, Maggie worked with Frank Gehry on the design of the Peter Lewis house. As Frank Gehry told me:

> Maggie was a good friend of mine. I knew her really well and I collaborated with her on a project that never got built, where she did the garden, and I did the house. I knew her well enough to know that she was not interested in Architecture.
>
> *(Gehry, 15.06.2018)*

In London, in a period of low activity, Maggie and Charles worked on the renovation of their house in Holland Park, the 'Thematic House', later renamed the aforementioned 'Cosmic House'. Appointing Terry Farrell as a project manager, Charles invited former AA students such as Piers Gough, Michael Graves, Rem Koolhaas and Jeremy Dixon to design one room each. As Piers told me "Of course, they all turned out strangely similar, i.e. 'Jencksian', except for Maggie's Jacuzzi designed as an inverted dome, which was all 'purest Gough'" (*15.05.2018*). Piers loved Maggie as much as anyone who knew her. "She was just absolutely divine and wonderful, outgoing and fun and generous". Always joyful, Maggie had an enormous amount of energy and, as her best friend Marcia Blakenham recalled, "she sort of brought light into a room" (BBC, 2016, 9:06).

In 1988, in Edinburgh, at the age of 47, Maggie was diagnosed with breast cancer. After seeing one oncologist after another, she underwent a mastectomy and began to recover. In 1994, however, after waiting in "this awful interior space with neon lights and sad people sitting exhausted on these chairs", she received the bad news that she only had two or three months left to live. Soon after this shocking 'death sentence', she was asked to leave the room, because the doctor had to see the next patient. *Where do you go? What can you do? Who can help you? Where can you have this time to adjust?* Traumatised, but mostly angry at the way she had been treated, Maggie lost hope. As Jencks recalled "she went home and I saw her curl up to die, she lost 20 pounds, turned white, she couldn't move". But, soon, something extraordinary happened. Probably driven by the natural instinct of attachment to life that we all have, encouraged by Charles' warning "if-you-must-die-you-better-do-it-by-fighting" Maggie decided to fight back. She wanted to give cancer patients a 'place' other than a windowless corridor so that no one would ever have the experience she had. Indeed, by waging this struggle, Maggie was able to help herself, and together with Charles underwent a mental transformation in which the memory of the healing temple of Asclepius returned, and Architecture and Health met.

The idea for this 'place' was born in a very modest way: a room at the end of the corridor of the Edinburgh hospital ward to be transformed into a pleasant environment "with a view onto nature, where one could sit peacefully between bouts of noxious therapy" (Jencks, 2015, p. 7). Maggie wanted to combat the lack of natural light, the fact that there was no view from her hospital bed, where, instead, there was a blinding neon light; the fact that the chairs were plastic and the bathroom doors didn't touch the ceiling or the floor "leaving her exposed and making her feel undignified" (*Maggie's@Salus, 2021*). Despite being an educated woman, she had realised that when someone, in a white coat, stood in front of her to give her bad news, she too felt tied up and was no longer able to understand, think or listen. Maggie wanted to change the attitude of the hospital which tells the patient: "In effect, how you feel is unimportant. You are not of value. Fit in with us, not us with you" into a "Welcome! And don't worry, we are here to reassure you, and your treatment will be good and helpful to you!" (Keswick, 1994, p. 21).

This is how the idea for a hospital room was quickly transformed into that of a centre outside the hospital, where cancer patients could wait for treatment away from the clinical environment, living moments of normal life. To find out which other similar facilities offered what she had in mind, Maggie asked her young nurse Laura Lee, fascinated by her ideas, to travel with her to California and explore the St.Monica Wellness Foundation hospice. Here, the two women discovered the benefits of good nutrition, exercise and comfort combined with a pleasant environment, coming to the conclusion that the new centre would not be clinical, but a place of practical, physical and psychological support. Back in Edinburgh, Maggie managed to raise £70,000 for her "CCC, Cancer Care Centre", persuading the hospital doctors to support her pilot idea and give her the abandoned stables Maggie used to see outside her bedroom window when she was admitted to the Oncology Unit.

After interviewing four architectural firms, Maggie and Charles commissioned Edinburgh-based Richard Murphy to renovate the small derelict in which to incorporate the "many things" (*Murphy, 11.06.2018*) that Maggie wanted to offer to people with cancer. What was absolutely clear from the start was that the centre had to be complementary to the hospital, but not institutional: no corridors, signs or information desks. "So, if the centre doesn't look like a hospital", Murphy wondered, "what is it?" The answer was that it had to be like a home, where the kitchen was at the heart for socialising over a cup of tea. Starting from the design idea of a double-height space with a single entrance and four rooms, Murphy managed, by raising the roof, to make two storeys, positioning the kitchen and the sitting room for various activities on the ground floor and the two consultation rooms on the first floor, obtaining flexible spaces suitable for multiple functions (Figure 3.2A and 3.2B).

For Murphy it was a priority to put people at ease, letting them in gradually, and allowing them to 'take' what was most convenient for them. Next to the kitchen was the wooden staircase, with two symmetrical flights, containing the aquarium that Maggie had requested and serving as a library with bookcases and seats, invited people to sit and read aloud but, at the same time, feel part of the scene (Figure 3.2C and 3.2D). With the exception of the bathroom door, which was completely closed "enough to cry without being heard" (Maggie's Brief, 2015, p. 8), Murphy had not provided doors in the building but sliding panels, so that the space could be divided in rooms or left open with absolute flexibility. Outside, a rose garden that was the horizon Maggie would have liked to see "amid attacks of harmful therapies" heralded the front door along with a sculpture, a bust of her by Charles' sister, artist Penelope Jencks. Thanks to her determination to follow Murphy's progress and develop the project, Maggie survived another 18 months.

Maggie Keswick Jencks died on July 8, 1995, at the age of 55, with drawings of her centre on her bed. At Maggie's funeral, Charles, Laura, Marcia and Richard Murphy knew that, after all the work they had done, the risk of failing to carry on Maggie's goal was very high, but, without hesitation, they all agreed that the plan was to continue. Although there was no formal document at the time, Maggie's Edinburgh—which opened in 1996 and was directed by Laura Lee—contained all of Maggie's ideas and wishes. Yet, as David Page recalls, the idea of writing an Architectural Brief was imminent.

> I remember how Maggie's Architectural Brief was born. It was in 1998, I think. It involved writing down the blueprint that Richard Murphy had done in an attempt to incorporate all of Maggie's ideas in Maggie's Edinburgh. The idea of writing a Brief was quite sudden and it was Charles, Laura and Marcia who wrote it. I remember it because it happened just before they interviewed me for Maggie's Infirmary. We were in a house in Glasgow, I think it was Laura's house.
>
> (*Page, 01.10.2018*)

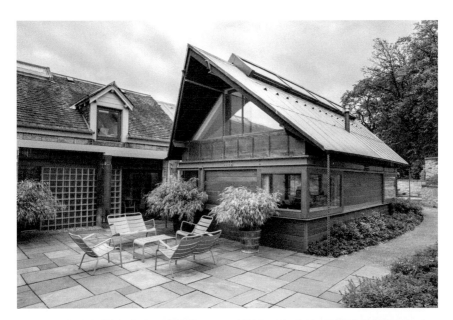

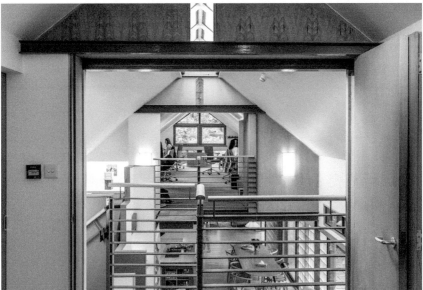

FIGURE 3.2A–3.2B   Maggie's Edinburgh (1996). View of the building as it appears today and of the kitchen on the ground floor glimpsed from the upper floor (©Marco Castelli Nirmal).

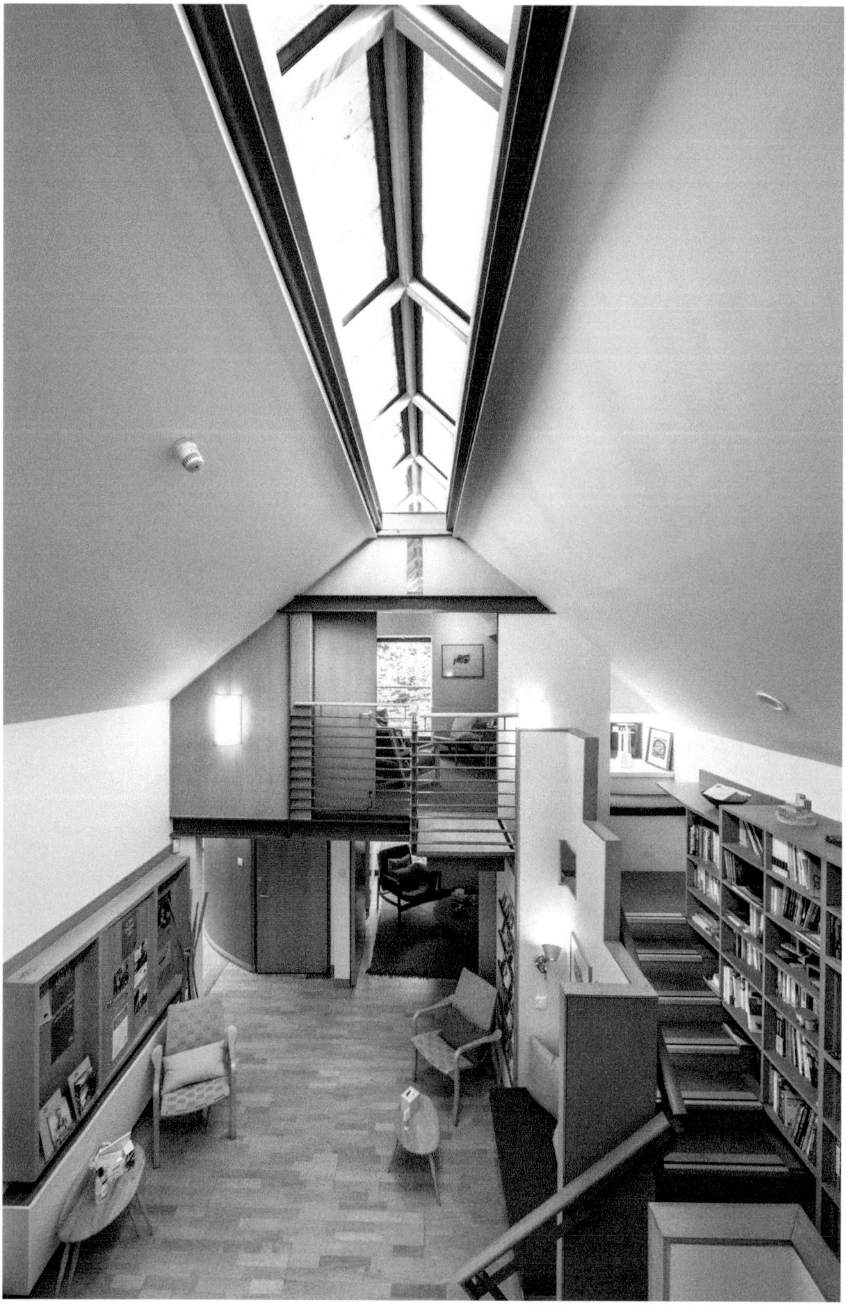

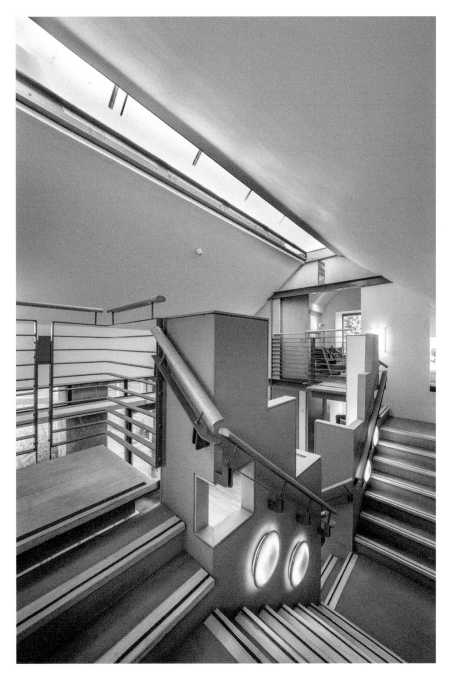

FIGURE 3.2C–3.2D   Maggie's Edinburgh (1996). View from above of the welcome area with the wooden staircase containing seating and bookcases (©Marco Castelli Nirmal).

Suddenly, the seed Maggie had planted began to grow. Knowing that Glasgow Cancer Hospital wanted one, Charles, Laura and Marcia asked David Page (Page\ Park), who had previously competed for the selection of the Edinburgh centre, to design it. After Page had completed Maggie's Glasgow the Gatehouse (2002) and Murphy had already doubled the size of Maggie's Edinburgh (2001), a new request for a third centre came from Ninewells Hospital in Dundee. This time it was not the conversion of an existing building, but a new building. Knowing how much Frank Gehry loved Maggie, Marcia suggested his name. Yet, when Maggie was alive and about to start her project, she had never asked Gehry to design it.

> Never. I knew she didn't want my design for her thing. She loved Charles Moore and Michael Graves and those people. So, it was strange to be asked to do it, afterwards. And I told him [Jencks]: 'she wouldn't want me to do it'.
>
> (*Gehry, 15.06.2018*)

But he did it. However, his early models—as he described them—were very 'sculptural' and 'active', too much for how he knew Maggie.

> And then I had a dream, one night, that she came to me and told me not to do that. So, I was very emotional, like I am now. I could cry again. So, I changed it. And I changed the building for something she would like. I knew what she wanted; it wasn't too fancy, it was more spatial, like this, nothing fancy. So, I made a lighthouse. And the lighthouse was for her to guide people in the darkness. And then I thought of the people, the view of the landscape looking down at the sea, the Firth of Tay. So, I thought 'you could go up in the tower and look at the Tay, and it will be quiet, it wouldn't be very active, it would be very serene, soft and not 'Architecture'. They need quiet. So, that's what I was doing.
>
> (*Gehry, 15.06.2018*)

Maggie's Dundee (2003) became a milestone in the charity's history. As it was Gehry's first building in the UK, his name immediately attracted the media who started talking about 'healing architecture'. In the past, Maggie and Charles were well aware of the role that 'design' and 'beauty' would play in healthcare. What even Charles Jencks had not predicted was how the Maggie's centre would be acclaimed in the world of architecture.

> We realised later that architecture put us on the map and since we have to raise all the money for our buildings, it made sense not to hide the fact that Frank Gehry designed it.
>
> (BBC, 2016, 32:12)

While it seemed that Jencks was aiming to hire famous architects, most of them were just old friends. In 2005, the already mentioned David Page (Page\Park) designed his second Maggie's centre in Inverness, Scottish Highlands. The following year, Zaha Hadid did Maggie's Fife (2006) and, shortly after, Ivan Harbour and

Richard Rogers (RSHP) were invited to design Maggie's West London (2008). Surprisingly enough, although the late Hadid was already world-famous by that time, like Gehry's building, Maggie's Fife was her first building in the UK. As for Harbour and Rogers, who despite being already known throughout the world for the Centre Pompidou in Paris and the Lloyds in London, their Maggie's centre was the first project in the office not to win a competition, but a simple commission.

From 2009 onwards, the opening of new centres has been exponential and, even today, despite the growing number of centres, the differences between one building and another are still considerable. As Jencks says in the BBC documentary on Maggie's (2016):

> Think of Maggie's as an experiment in a Petri dish, where you put different ingredients, the same programme, but out-pop all these completely different buildings, and they are all good solutions! In mathematics and in most professions, you can't have twenty different answers, and all be correct, but with Architecture, it's interesting that you can have that pluralism of response.
>
> (BBC, 2016, 34:55)

Today there are thirty Maggie's centres in the world, mainly in the United Kingdom, but new centres are under construction or in the planning stages and more and more hospitals are asking for one, and more and more architects are offering to design one.

Maggie's Legacy and Organisation

Architecture is organisation. You are a organiser, not a drawing board stylist.
(Le Corbusier, 'Focus' 1, 1938)

The establishment of the "Maggie Keswick Jencks Cancer Caring Trust" (the official name of the Maggie's centre) in 1995 and the rapid expansion of the charity in the UK and overseas demonstrated the strength of Maggie's original concept and the need of local communities for this new type of healthcare facility. Coming to London, with the construction of Maggie's West London at Charing Cross Hospital in 2008 as the first centre outside Scotland, represented the ultimate growth of the organisation and the beginning of a different kind of care.

London was unlike any previous site and there was a lot of uncertainty about which route to take. As Laura Lee recalls: "No one knew really what we had to do, so we had to establish ourselves as an organisation" (BBC, 2016, 35:48). While the centre was under construction, the new branch settled in a small space loaned by Richard Rogers above the River Café in Hammersmith, to move to its current office nearby a few years later. Instead, when Glasgow's second centre, Maggie's Gartnavel (2011), was built, the former Maggie's Glasgow the Gatehouse (2002) became Maggie's office for Scotland.

Today, Maggie's is an independent organisation where Dame Laura Lee is the Chief Executive Officer and Queen Consort Camilla is the President. Maggie's is governed by the Board of Directors and carried out by the Executive Group and the Architecture Co–Clients. The latter—today represented by Laura Lee and Marcia Blakenham after the death of Charles Jencks in 2019—are responsible for commissioning projects, following those in progress and creating future ones. In total, 280 administrative and centre staff members in the UK and 24 people in the rest of the world worked for the organisation in 2022. To these numbers we must add that of all the volunteers, including those who raise funds. In this regard, Maggie's does not receive government funding, but relies on the generosity of local communities and different types of donors.

In terms of fund management, what Maggie's does differently from other healthcare facilities is letting its donors know, in full transparency, how the money is being used. As confirmed by Maggie's visitors, this is very important to them, because knowing where the money goes helps people with cancer feel in good hands.

> Two years ago, when Sue died, we wanted to make a donation, but someone said 'whatever you do, don't sign the check to just the Marie Curie, make it out to Marie Curie Hampstead Hospice, because if it goes to the head office, Hampstead won't see it'. This is what happens with the big charities. And this is what is so nice about Maggie's, because you know that if you donate anything here, it will go here, for management or staff and offices.
>
> *(Focus-group Barts)*

The Maggie's centre is open from 9am to 5pm—sometimes even until 9pm—from Monday to Friday. The staff team varies according to the size of the centre, but the basic figures are essentially three clinical (Centre Head, Psychologist and Cancer Support Specialist [CCS]) and two non-clinical (Benefit Advisor and Fundraiser). All of Maggie's permanent staff have a hospital background, especially CSS who have experience as oncology or radiology nurses. Among the temporary staff, there are many types of volunteers (full-time or part-time) who had relatives or were themselves people with cancer now in remission. While it is mainly volunteers who welcome newcomers with greetings and the tea ceremony, a strong sense of hospitality is required of all staff, regardless of their precise role.

As for the relationship with the hospital, it has evolved over time. At the beginning, there was the firm belief that the Maggie's centre was complementary but not institutional, therefore the opposite of the hospital.

> At the time of the planning application, it was very important to Maggie's that we didn't put a lift in the building. Lifts were seen as institutional. Anything that seems institutional is an anathema to Maggie's, and I can understand that. So, they would say 'we wouldn't have a lift in a house, we will never have a lift'. But, of course, in legal terms, in a non-residential 'house' you have to provide a lift for accessibility purposes, otherwise you do not meet building control

requirements. The most difficult things were negotiating for an exemption and ensuring the centre didn't have to install a means of escape sign, saying 'escape out of the back'. They are small things, but they are actually, bureaucratically massive, and they mean a huge amount to what, the perception of the building not being an institution but actually just being a lovely place to feel, help you feel good.

(Harbour, 20.07.2018)

Today, Maggie's organisation avoids opposing the hospital and, although it was so important to Charles Jencks to say "we are a contrast", today it works closely with local NHS trusts to bring support to as many parts of the UK as possible. "Our ambition is to be at 50% of all major NHS hospitals in the UK by 2022" (Maggie's Professionals, 2023). Although it might seem a step back from Maggie's original philosophy, this new position of collaboration shows a sign of maturity in line with the future model of healthcare cooperation that I will explain in Chapter 7.

How the Architecture Supports Maggie's

At Maggie's, the support that architecture provides to the organisation is reflected in the way staff assist visitors. Once visitors are heard entering, thanks to the open view from the kitchen, the staff is able to understand if visitors are new, and need immediate help, or if they are old users, and know what they are looking for. In this, architecture helps tell people which direction to take.

The curiosity of the scheme is that as soon as you enter, you want to walk through the space. The building is a sequence of different types of spaces, and that is a kind of curiosity.

(van Loon, 16.05.2018)

At Maggie's Glasgow, the design idea is that the more the building is exposed to the landscape, the more social the space is; the further the building goes into the forest, the more private the rooms become. The front door, midway and central to the building, is visible from everywhere, from the kitchen, from the office area across the garden and from the group activity room. Thus conceived, the building certainly does not need CCT cameras to support the staff who, with great discretion, know how to be present while keeping an eye on visitors in other areas of the building (Figure 3.3).

I was surprised with Maggie's, because making a building for that function is one thing but deciding how to manage it is another matter entirely. So, it's not just about the architecture, but the way the staff manage it. The combination of all of this is a crucial part of the success of this centre.

(van Loon, 15.05.2018)

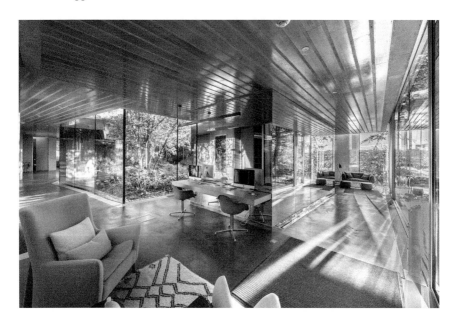

FIGURE 3.3 Maggie's buildings support the staff who, with great discretion, know how to be present while keeping an eye on visitors (Maggie's Glasgow, 2011) (©Marco Castelli Nirmal).

Leaving staff to take the lead in supporting Maggie's visitors, the layout of the rooms and their content is left to the co–clients Laura and Marcia, and nothing is left to chance. Despite the apparent normality of the domestic setting, Maggie's has precise rules that I only learned after spending a few months there. In fact, what is allowed and what is not allowed is not so obvious. For example, only a certain type of kettle can be used, microwave ovens and clocks are forbidden, there is no air conditioning, towels can only be terrycloth and the furnishings are both traditional and highly sought after in design. "Really? How strange?" In reality, it is not strange at all, because it means that Maggie's organisation cares and, in this, the staff must understand the importance of 'design' and 'beauty' in triggering the therapeutic process.

> What happens here is that the building entirely supports, because the building is holding in everything: in the views to the horizon, in the light, in the space, and the furniture. It's saying: 'I'm going to make this as nice as possible for you at a time where that's probably as horrible as possible for you'.
>
> (*Psychologist Dundee*)

> No matter where people look, they're always seeing something that is pleasing. And I think that helps, and I think maybe in a more unconscious way. And even today, after 16 years I have been coming here every day, no matter where I am in this building, I always look and see something that's different, you are

always surprised. I don't think when people are coming in, they take the building for granted, they are warmed by it and welcomed by it. I am a professional nurse and I probably don't know how to speak about architecture, but I think that is the beauty of architecture, it's the fact that someone can actually design something that increases feelings. It's soothing, it's pleasing and uplifting and quirky and gay.

(CCS_no.2 Dundee)

In terms of spaces dedicated to the staff, the Architectural Brief does not foresees a 'staff room' or any separation between staff and visitors in the building, because their coexistence and collaboration is what triggers the therapeutic process. Indeed, as stated by psychologist and neuroscientist Sabina Brennan, who at the time of the interview directed a dementia research programme at Trinity College Dublin, in healthcare 'integration' is a priority. Interviewed by Níall McLaughlin and Yeoryia Manolopoulou as part of their research on dementia conducted in preparation of the Alzheimer Respite Centre project in Dublin (2011) exhibition at the 2016 Venice Biennale of Architecture (Losing Myself, 2016), the psychologist argues that providing an organisation with a "staff station" means characterising it with "segregation", stating that staff treat patients as something 'less' or 'other'.

It's what I call the 'othering', they are different. So why are you eating somewhere else? Shouldn't we eat together? If you have a caregiver in your house that caregiver has dinner with you, that caregiver prepares dinner and you eat together!

(Brennan, 2015, 45:30)

While this may seem like a lack of support towards the staff, not including the staff station in a design brief means designing spaces that respond to the needs of all people with the ultimate goal of generating an ideal and caring community, from which both patients and staff will benefit (Brennan, 2015). In the UK healthcare sector this never happens; there is no circumstance, in fact, in which the staff does not have their own 'sluice' or 'staff station' which, in a hospital design brief, is an indisputable requirement. The fact that the Architectural Brief does not require a 'staff station' and instead offers open spaces, inviting staff and visitors to come together around the kitchen table, is what sets Maggie's apart from all other organisations.

Maggie's Support Programme and Life at the Centre

Maggie's current support programme is the result of improvements made over many years. As reported by Charles Jencks (2015), among the strategies that Maggie adopted to react to the 'death sentence' received in hospital, there were ten actions that she called "guerrilla tactics": yoga, Tai chi and Qigong exercises, relaxation and Ayurvedic therapy to lower her level of psychological stress; counselling with psychologists and Vipassana meditation to deal with her family problems; Chinese herbs, capsules of mushrooms and vitamins for her physical benefit. Maggie's Chinese background certainly came through in her choice of oriental and complementary/natural therapies.

Of all the actions she had taken, however, Maggie's most effective strategy was to change her diet, which had an empowering psychological impact. As Charles explained to me, acting immediately, regaining control, and getting something rewarding for herself was what gave Maggie the will to fight by any means possible. Indeed, in the conclusions of *A View from the Front Line* (1994), Charles had urged Maggie to use the phrase "empower the patient". In doing so, Maggie realised that for a cancer patient, the secret to navigate through many choices "down here in the war zone" was "self-help" (Jencks, 2015, p. 20), an active involvement in one's own therapy. And becoming the spokesperson for her experience with cancer in an effort to help others react and fight their own battles, Maggie left behind another vital aspect that gave birth to her programme: the paradox of the liberating therapy of struggle and humour evident in the cheering quote that describes her last year as "The best year of my life" (Jencks, 2015, p. 13).

Today, Maggie's guerrilla tactics have become the basis of a programme whose original three areas of *Lifestyle, Emotional* and *Practical* support have been significantly expanded (Appendix II). The offer of support is similar in all centres, but it's not exactly the same, depending on several factors such as instructor availability, user demand and, of course, local culture and traditions. The courses are held on a weekly or monthly basis and by session or appointment. For a better understanding, see the list of activities offered in the three types of support that were going on at Maggie's Dundee, Maggie's Oldham and Maggie's Barts in 2019, during my ethnographic work (Frisone, 2021).

Of the three types of support offered, the *Lifestyle* is the one that includes the activities that concern the 'body', i.e. physical, nutritional, creative-manual, while the *Emotional* is the one that includes the activities that concern the emotions and the 'mind'. However, because at Maggie's mind and body are connected, the combination of the two types of support will go beyond their primary goals. Within the *Emotional* support, the "Architecture, Art, Landscape and Flowers" category is perhaps the most immediate for visitors to understand how Maggie's environment helps support people's emotions. In particular, the friendly and convivial atmosphere of the aforementioned 'kitchenism' (i.e. how Jencks called Maggie's welcoming ritual made up of a cup of tea and lots of colored cushions that warm hands and heart), along with the unconventional architecture that welcomes people into cosy areas to sit and observe art and nature, are of primary importance and value. Usually, unconventionality tends to be poorly understood. However, at Maggie's, it serves to intrigue and distract visitors and makes them appreciate its purpose when applied to architecture. Over time, in fact, people with cancer become familiar with the space and begin to understand the relationship between the building and their experience, which architectural features make them feel good and why (Figure 3.4).

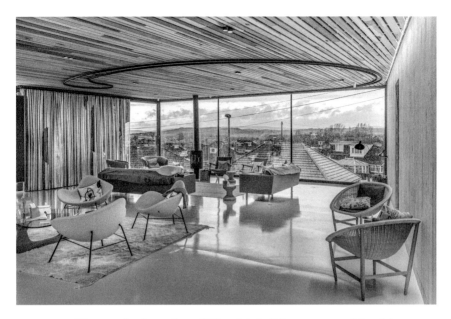

FIGURE 3.4 The open horizon view of Maggie's buildings supports Maggie's strategy of "empowering the patient" (Maggie's Oldham, 2017) (©Marco Castelli Nirmal).

> The design of this building is so relaxing, it's like the Scandinavian one. I mean, you haven't got a brick wall they're happy with; they want you to have a nice view.
>
> (*Focus-group Oldham*)

This fact is facilitated by the presence of many books on architecture which, on the shelves of Maggie's libraries, sit alongside those on cancer. As Jencks (2015) recounts, to understand everything about her disease Maggie read a lot and her favorite text was *Options: The Alternative Cancer Therapy Book* by Richard Walters, which was subtitled 'For people who want to make informed decisions about alternative treatments against cancer'. Indeed, within the *Practical* support, another important offering of the programme is the 'Information for visitors and families', which Maggie used to define as 'power', but only if supported by the knowledge of "what it means" (Keswick, 1994). With their limitations, patients can be good diagnosticians, and that's why Maggie's makes available to visitors, in addition to books, computer stations to be able to do in-depth research into their disease.

Arriving at Maggie's for the First Time

The ways and circumstances in which visitors come to Maggie's for the first time vary. From the moment they receive the diagnosis, it is usually a matter of days, sometimes hours, before people visit the centre, depending on who suggested going to Maggie's. They may have been not only doctors or nurses in the hospital or secretaries from other cancer centres like Macmillan, but also friends who have had the same experience with cancer. These moments, in which "a diagnosis hits like a bomb that destroys a person's plans and dreams in terms of career, education, sense of self, body image, finances and practicality" (Howells, 2016), represent 'traumatic transitions', which manifest themselves through the transformation of the way the brain organises perceptions. In an attempt to convey to the reader the strong emotional state a patient experiences when receiving a cancer diagnosis, I recommend watching Maggie's short video entitled "Breathing Space" (Maggie's Videos, 2019).

> Trauma, by definition, is unbearable and intolerable. (…) While all of us would like to 'go beyond' trauma, the part of our brain responsible for ensuring survival (located well below the rational brain) is not so good as to deny. (…) Feeling that they are not in control of themselves, traumatised people live in a state of persistent fear.
>
> (Van der Kolk, 2015, pp. 3–4)

Having experienced it personally, I can say that trauma not only changes what you think and the way you think, but also your actual ability to think. To overcome it and for a real change to occur, it is necessary that both brain and body, together, know that the worst is over and that they live in the present moment or, if the danger is still ongoing, that the place where the post–trauma is lived is safe and is there to protect you (Van der Kolk, 2015).

To live in the present moment, we must try not to relive past traumatic emotions embedded in the 'memory records' of 'dispositions', we create. Borrowing from Eberhard (2009), explaining what Damasio (1999, cited in Eberhard, 2009) means by 'dispositional representations' or simply 'dispositions', using the example of a 'good' memory record, I wish to attempt to use a 'bad' memory record to explain to the reader what happens in the cancer patient's brain if these dispositions or recordings of "dormant and implicit" memories resurface. These recordings lie just below the surface of consciousness and include (1) our perception of an object (e.g., a chair in the doctor's office who gave us the diagnosis), (2) the sensory aspects of that object (colour, shape, texture) and (3) the motor regulations that accompanied the collection of sensory signals and the emotional reactions of the painful body state we had towards the object (when we sat on the chair and listened to the doctor's voice).

Once a disposition is recorded, the day we return to a doctor's office and see that chair—or a similar one—our brain will retrieve that disposition along with previously stored related information and will remember not only our sensory experience of that visit, but also the emotional reactions of the past (Damasio, 1999, cited in Eberhard, 2009). This emotional experience, which manifests in the body through sweating or the acceleration of the heartbeat, takes place in the prefrontal cortices of the brain, which are ideal for participation in reasoning and decision-making because they are connected to every chemical and motor response pathway available to the brain. This demonstrates the importance of visceral information in the cognitive process (Damasio, 1994). Once the body has repaired itself and knows it is safe, it communicates it to the brain and the brain will release relief and reduce all the physical manifestations of the emotional experience, in this case fear. This is where the Maggie's centre comes into play which, thanks to its welcoming architecture, will give the brain the information and the feeling of 'safety'. In designing a healthcare environment, since the nervous system responses of traumatised individuals are more sensitive (Van der Kolk, 2015), the architect must know that the sensory input must come from a connected and fully celebrated place (Erwine, 2016).

Three to five new visitors arrive at Maggie's every day. As previously described, as soon as they enter, the staff is ready at the door to greet them with a welcoming smile and a metaphorical hug. Usually accompanied by family members—because, unlike the hospital from which they are excluded for privacy reasons, Maggie's includes families—new visitors are greeted in the welcome area, which is located near the door to reassure them that they can leave at any time, and where they will be offered tea in a real ceramic cup and not in a plastic one like in the hospital. From here, as we know, the first space that visitors see—which is unusual for a healthcare facility—is the kitchen. Seeing it spacious and full of people busy preparing food and drinks, newcomers immediately experience a sense of familiarity and even relief. As they observe people laughing or conversing despite their illness, they instantly feel in tune with the environment (Figure 3.5).

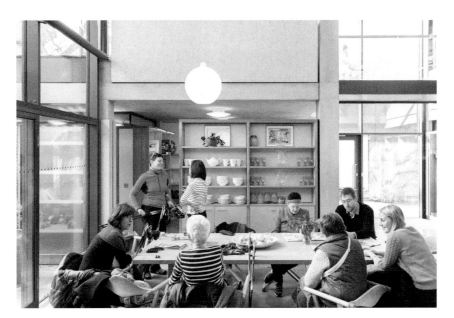

FIGURE 3.5   The first space that visitors arriving at Maggie's see is the kitchen. Seeing it spacious and full of people busy preparing food and drinks, newcomers immediately feel a sense of familiarity (Maggie's West London, 2008) (Courtesy of Maggie's).

How It Works

On the notice board, visitors can find the schedule for the courses that take place at the centre every day, five days a week. These are of different types and whether the visitor chooses one depends the support they are looking for. If they want to attend yoga, nutrition or art therapy (all *Lifestyle* support), without booking, visitors arrive shortly before the course starts. For example, if the course starts at 10am, people will arrive around 9:45am and immediately prepare coffee and tea for themselves and their family or friends. At 10am, the busy kitchen suddenly empties out to become a quiet space with maybe just a couple of people, while the large sitting room is transformed into the group activity room that will remain in use until the centre closes at 5pm and sometimes later.

At the end of each activity, the kitchen fills up again, especially during the lunch break, when the staff often dine sharing the kitchen table with visitors. After a quiet moment of coffee and a chat, around 1pm new visitors arrive to attend the afternoon activities. The last visitors arrive between 4pm and 5pm or later if some courses such as choir or move-dance-feel—but only in some centres—are scheduled between 5pm and 9pm. For those who don't come to attend a course but only for a 'cup of tea and biscuits', by themselves or in company, most visits depend on the treatment appointments. This type of visitor arrives at any time of the day and their stay can last the time between one appointment and another or even longer if they stop at the end of the day, before returning home.

Visitors who have booked an individual psychological session—which usually takes place in one of the two consultation rooms—will spend their waiting time before the meeting in the welcome area, where the building will intervene to distract and reassure them. As Maggie Keswick has argued, during doctor visits the environment is of the utmost importance.

> Waiting time could be used positively. Sitting in a pleasant, but by no means expensive room, with thoughtful lighting, a view out to trees, birds and sky, and chairs and sofas arranged in various groupings could be an opportunity for patients to relax and talk, away from home cares.
>
> (Keswick, 1994, p. 21)

Thanks to the experience of waiting, new visitors to Maggie's gradually begin to observe the building and its architecture and to understand the difference between this place and the spaces they were used to. Realising that they are in a place "never seen before", in this phase, their point of reference is still the staff members. Indeed, according to Charles Jencks, it is the programme together with the spirit of the staff that makes the difference in Maggie's success and constitutes the common thread between all the centres, which allow for the same feelings. For him, architecture and art have an indirect effect on people with cancer, first passing through the staff: "Architecture supports the staff who in turn supports the patients" (Jencks, 2012, p. 37). It is true that, in general, if employees enjoy their work, they will treat customers better. However, as we will see later, the architecture has a direct impact on all users, staff and visitors, and what unites the centres derives not only from the same type of work carried out by the staff, but also from something else, which I will explain in Chapter 5.

Maggie's Buildings

The non-clinical Maggie's centre is always located on the hospital grounds, integrating the clinical activity while maintaining its distinctive identity. The site, usually a former car park lot or brownfield area near the Oncology Unit, offered free by the hospital, can vary depending on the situation. As a result of this morphological variety—but also thanks to the open and free interpretation of the Architectural Brief left to the architects—both the landscape and the architecture of Maggie's centres are very different from each other, even if, as Maggie's claims, each centre contributes to its mission by generating the same psychological effects in people (*Howells, 2017*).

With an average total area of 300–450 m², depending on the reference cancer population, the Maggie's centre is a small building that stands out for its visual impact or is hidden in a luxuriant garden; once located, the building is inviting, and the entrance encourages people to enter. "It is the invitation that is incredibly important" (*Blackenham, 18.05.2019*). In fact, as the Brief requires, the building must amuse, stimulate, intrigue, make people smile and lift their spirits. From this point of view, among the centres, some are more or less iconic than others, considering 'iconic' a positive term (Figure 3.6).

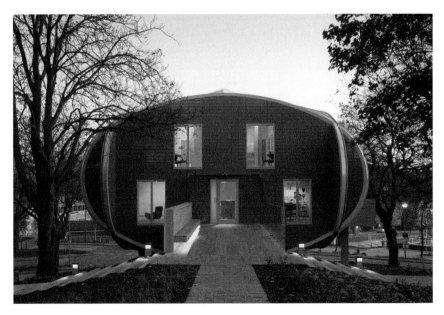

FIGURE 3.6   Among the centres, some are more iconic than others. The iconic facade entertains and makes you smile (Maggie's Nottingham, 2011) (©Martine Hamilton Knight).

Iconic or not iconic? Like Piers's, I just think it's amusing and light-hearted and it makes you smile and fun. Or Rem Koolhaas's is enticing. There is something about his building that is curious. And we are talking about feelings and what feelings that building engenders. Literally, when you walk through the door, it's extraordinary. 'But when you see it in the landscape, you are curious about it. You wonder 'Oh I wonder what it is'. So, you are still attracted, but in a different way. Neither way is wrong, as long as you have been led in a way'.

(Lee and Blackenham, 18.05.2019)

Once inside, the absence of typical hospital corridors and, conversely, the presence of open and semi–open spaces derived by the design principle of 'spatial interaction rather than walls' allows for an immediate understanding of the building's layout and, as seen, encourages movement. The openness of the spaces also implies the closeness of the different conversations made possible by the relaxed attitude of the users and by some differences in level and smaller spaces within the larger space which guarantee distance and intimacy. In response to the Brief's call for openness and continuity, as mentioned, the doors are designed to be intentionally left open, so they slide or rotate, which helps people forget to close them and not worry about privacy. "At Maggie's, very little happens behind closed doors" (*Howells, 16.06.2017*).

Architecture

In the last pages of the concise Architectural Brief (2015), we can find a short explanation of the few functional requirements that the reader may recognise in the floor plan of Maggie's Glasgow Gartnavel (Figure 3.7) (For floorplans of the other centres see Appendix IV). These functions can be very flexibly adapted to the three different types of support, *Lifestyle, Emotional* and *Practical,* and are all suitable for welcoming newcomers: the welcome area and the library lend themselves mainly to *Practical* support; the kitchen and large sitting or group activity room primarily accommodate *Lifestyle* support; consultation rooms house the *Emotional* support. Among other functions necessary to facilitate visitors and make the organisation work, there are also the small office area and the car park.

Entrance/'Pause'

As the Architectural Brief states, "the entrance should be obvious, welcoming, and not intimidating, with a place to hang your coat and leave your brolly. The door should not be draughty, so perhaps there should be a lobby". Although described as an interior, the 'pause' space—which did not once exist—throughout my ethnographic work has felt more like an exterior space, which over time has become increasingly important for inviting people into the building, giving them the time and freedom to choose whether to enter or not and possibly try again next time. In

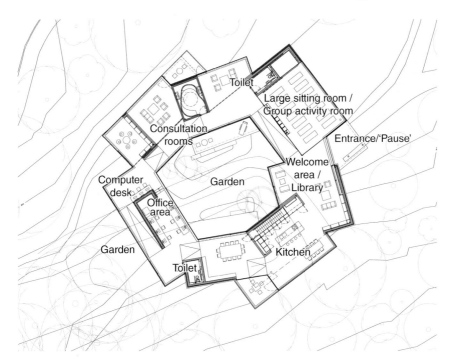

FIGURE 3.7 Floorplan of Maggie's Glasgow (2011) with the few functional requirements of the Architectural Brief (Courtesy of OMA).

fact, some visitors have told me that they made several attempts before being able
to enter the building the first time, and the 'pause' space outside the building gave
them time to decide (Figure 3.8). Differently interpreted by the architects, for
Darron Haylock (Foster+Partners) the idea of the 'pause' space at Maggie's Manchester (2016), where to meditate and "feel protected from the typical Manchester
rain", is a veranda—like an American porch—overlooking the lush nature at the
entrance to the building, where people can sit and feel strong enough to enter (*Haylock, 12.06.2018*) (Figure 3.9). For Ivan Harbour, the 'pause' space was interpreted
as a sequence of steps (Figure 3.10).

> Yes, the door had to be obvious, but Maggie's did say they wanted a 'pause'.
> And this was something I found intriguing and it led to the idea that the ap-
> proach would be a series of thresholds. So, you can wait here, you can see
> where you're going to go, but you don't have to make that move until you are
> comfortable. This is a big moment for anyone coming to the centre. You have an
> opportunity to pause before you come in. It's about pausing, so this is why these
> thresholds were absolutely critical, they gave you time, some distance to reflect
> and you felt that this was a positive.
>
> (*Harbour, 20.07.2018*)

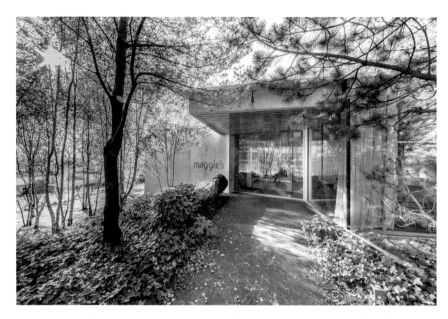

FIGURE 3.8 Before entering, Maggie's buildings give you time to decide. The 'pause' space could be a simple tree trunk where you can sit and meditate (Maggie's Glasgow, 2011) (©Marco Castelli Nirmal).

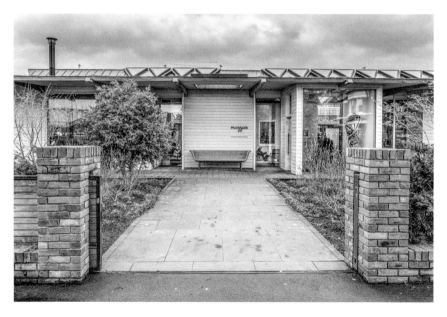

FIGURE 3.9 The 'pause' space can also be a veranda like an American porch (Maggie's Manchester, 2016) (©Marco Castelli Nirmal).

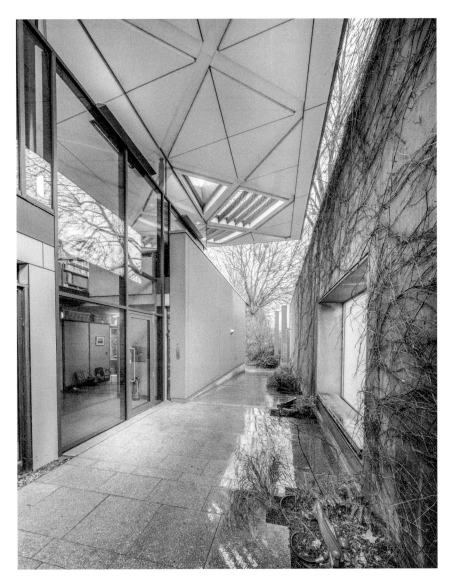

FIGURE 3.10 The 'pause' space can be a series of thresholds (Maggie's West London, 2008) (©Marco Castelli Nirmal).

The moment experienced by new visitors in the 'pause' space is very complex due to the myriad emotions they can feel while looking at the door of the building. Establishing a first contact with the newcomers, at Maggie's the front door is essential to convince them to enter, just as in history doors have always been a symbol of the passage between two worlds, a fact that even neuroscientists understand now.

It took me a long time to understand why the architect André Bruyère was so interested in doors, but now it is obvious to me. The door is one of the most important elements in architecture, experienced as a front for emotions, fading actions, and the construction of memories.

(Berthoz, 2000, p. 259)

Welcome Area/Library

Upon entering a Maggie's centre, visitors will access the welcome area/library. As the Architectural Brief states, "the first impression must be encouraging. There should be somewhere for you and a friend or relative to sit, a shelf with some books and an ability to assess, more or less, the layout of the rest of the building". As previously mentioned, the welcome area is a space, as bright as possible, with an open view towards the space inside and, at the same time, towards nature outside. Here there are no reception desks of typical health facilities, nor signage of any kind (plates on doors, badges on uniforms, orientation signs), but only coloured armchairs that evoke a familiar atmosphere; a notice board that tells the activities that take place in the centre is also located here or in the kitchen (Figure 3.11). Originally combined with the library to help visitors, while waiting, to overcome the difficulties of the moment by reading a book or a brochure, this is no longer always the case, and the library can be further away from the front door, resulting in a quieter space for visitors who can isolate themselves while remaining in sonar contact with the rest of the centre.

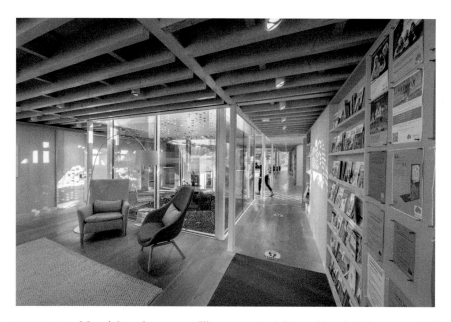

FIGURE 3.11 Maggie's welcome area/library greets visitors with colorful seats, a shelf filled with brochures and books and a notice board describing the centre's activities (Maggie's Lanarkshire, 2014) (©Marco Castelli Nirmal).

Kitchen

Maggie's kitchen, even when it rains, is always bright and warm (Figure 3.12). As required by the Architectural Brief, like a 'country' kitchen, it "should have room

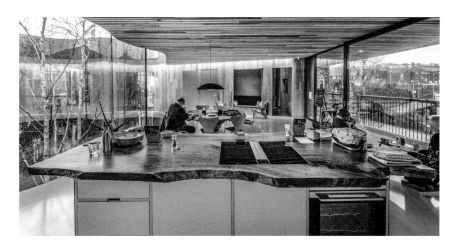

FIGURE 3.12   Maggie's kitchen, even when it rains, is always bright and warm (Maggie's Oldham, 2017) (©Marco Castelli Nirmal).

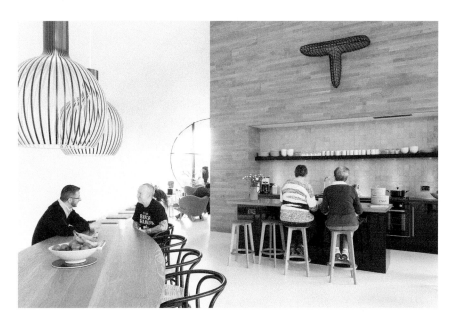

FIGURE 3.13   Different in each centre, the kitchen table can take any shape. At Maggie's Aberdeen (2017) it is oval (Courtesy of Maggie's).

for a large table for 12 people" that can also be used for demonstrations/seminars/ groups discussion. Different in each centre, the large table—which inevitably draws people in difficult situations to it and facilitates their opening process—can take any shape. Oblong tables, for example, work well because they give the possibility of having several conversations at the same table. Indeed, at Maggie's Aberdeen the table is oval, because Snøhetta thinks that "a long rectangular table would not work the same way. But we also believe that round tables invite more people to sit" (*Aabø, 02.11.2018*) (Figure 3.13). A unique feature of the Maggie's centre, the kitchen table is considered by the visitors to be a fundamental tool, "the pedal to start the day".

Consultation Rooms

The consultation rooms are of two sizes, a medium-sized one for group conversations of up to 12 people, with a fireplace or stove to create a more convivial atmosphere (Figure 3.14), and a smal-sized one for individual consultations. As described by the Architectural Brief, "they should have some character and maybe have sliding doors to become a second large room, which can be left open and inviting when not in use". The first room will be used for small workshops and

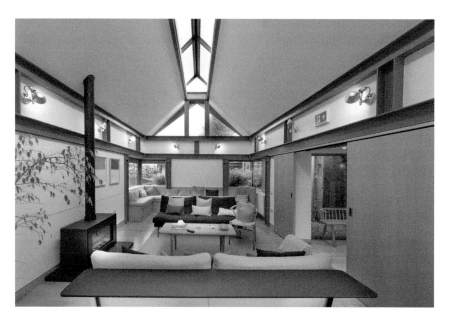

FIGURE 3.14   Medium-sized consultation rooms can accommodate groups of up to 12 people, welcoming them with a fireplace to create a more convivial environment (Maggie's Edinburgh, 2018 addition) (©Marco Castelli Nirmal).

sessions, while the second, for just two people, will be used for confidential conversations with in–house psychologists or external professionals such as oncologists and financial experts. These rooms always have windows that look outwards, towards nature or towards the sky, comfortable chairs that can be moved around, warm blankets and colourful pillows. The Staff told me that people can sit next to them and not in front of them, so as to avoid the interlocutor's gaze and instead look outside, which helps to open up and start a conversation.

Large Sitting Room or Group Activity Room

As requested by the Brief, the large sitting room "offers enough space to accommodate 14 people lying down and a storage room for folding chairs and yoga mats. As much as possible, you should be able to open and shut walls (perhaps between this and welcome area/kitchen area) to have flexi-space, for more or less privacy, as occasion demands. The relaxation space should be capable of being soundproof when closed off". Warm and welcoming, the large sitting room, furnished with comfortable armchairs, beautiful carpets, warm light lamps and artwork, becomes a group activity room and, depending on the activity, becomes a room for *Emotional* support (relaxation, mindfulness, cancer groups), physical and dynamic *Lifestyle* support (Tai chi, yoga, move-more) or social *Lifestyle* support (choir, beauty, conferences, fundraising meetings) (Figure 3.15). Visitors I met identified the group activity room as 'work' and 'action' as opposed to the kitchen which they saw as 'fun' and 'relax'.

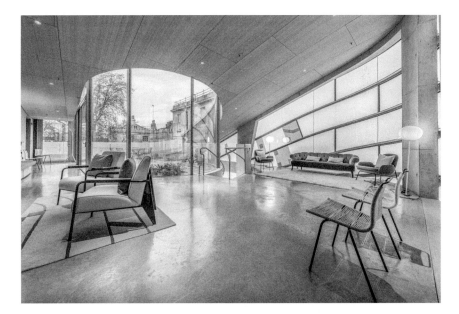

FIGURE 3.15   At Maggie's the large sitting room, furnished with comfortable armchairs, beautiful carpets, and warm light lamps transforms flexibly into a group activity room (Maggie's Barts, 2017) (©Marco Castelli Nirmal).

Toilets

Long called 'private' in England, the toilet is a very private room, where visitors can face the most difficult moments, such as bad news or mourning, and cry without being heard. For this, the toilet must be completely closed and not have gaps above and below the door as in the hospital. Of the two required, at least one must be large enough to accommodate a chair and a bookshelf.

Art

At Maggie's, art is as important as architecture, because it helps visitors and staff see the world from a different point of view. "Hanging a work of art is like opening a window: it gives you a view. And you look at it and you are enchanted. It is not a decoration" (*Blakenham, 18.05.2019*) (Figure 3.16). The acquisition of works of art in Maggie's centres was made possible thanks to the donation of artists such as Maggie and Charles' old Scottish friend, Edoardo Paolozzi and many others who have contributed to enriching the MAG (Maggie's Art Group) collection. Because it contains a large number of works of art, the Maggie's centre can now be described as a 'place of art', reinforcing Jencks' hybrid concept. In healthcare, being a place of art is a quite rare if not unique condition. However, some hospitals have started to place 'hospital art' in waiting rooms and corridors, even though, in general, specialists who design interior spaces in the healthcare sector do not consider art and the aesthetic experience a priority.

This experience has been the subject of many studies in Neuroesthetics, which has concluded that "there can be no satisfactory theory of aesthetics that is not

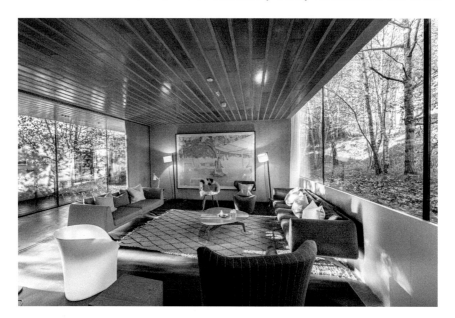

FIGURE 3.16   At Maggie's, hanging a work of art is like opening a window, it gives you a view (Maggie's Glasgow, 2011) (©Marco Castelli Nirmal).

neurobiological based" (Zeki, 2001, quoted in Mallgrave, 2013, p. 33). Even Darwin, at a certain point in his research, had intuited that *beauty* was an important parameter, so much so that he added it to his work *On the Origin of Species* (1859), which later became *The Descendent of Man* (1874). After a long period of disinterest, as Mallgrave (2013) explains, *beauty* has returned to the spotlight and, more recently, fMRI (functional magnetic resonance imaging) investigations have revealed that "there is something neurologically tangible to the aesthetic experience that we define as beautiful" (2013, p. 21). Although throughout history artists have always known that *beauty* was a weapon of 'conquest' and painters such as Cézanne, Malevič, Mondrian, Van Gogh knew that using only lines or shapes or certain colours or "exaggerating" with unconventional schemes sent stimuli to the observer that "provoke the brain with enigmas and striking visual expressions" (2013, p. 34), it is only today that we understand the physiological connection between art and the organism, and that pleasure is "preeminently an emotional experience as well as one that is chemically induced" (2013, p. 34), which has benefits on our brain and body.

The artistic *beauty* of Kálida Barcelona (2019) lies in the floral motifs of its roofing and facade cladding, which in turn are inspired by the motifs and colours of the ceramics used in the nearby Hospital de la Santa Creu I Sant Pau (1902–1930), a masterpiece of Catalan modernist architecture. As Benedetta Tagliabue recounts, according to her husband Enric Miralles, who had shown her the hospital—"one of the pieces he loved most"—as soon as she arrived in Barcelona, Domènech i Montaner had really created a very social project here, in which "beauty works to make people feel healthier" (*Tagliabue, 19.11.2018*).

In search of 'neuronal correlates' of *beauty*, today, neuroscientists have discovered that the sensory signals that reach the nerves of the retina, and which, through the optic nerve, reach the occipital lobe (the one at the base of the head that deals with the vision processing), are subdivided—and never recomposed again—into categories relating to different areas (lines, shapes, colours and movement), which process data simultaneously but at different speeds as "colour, for instance, being perceived before form or motion" (Zeki and Bartles, 1999, cited in Mallgrave, 2013, p. 40). This explains why, at Maggie's, colour is so regarded and used.

In addition to the artwork acquired by artists who were old friends of the Jencks, at Maggie's, every architect who designs a centre is committed to involving local artists along with those from their own country. For example, at Maggie's Aberdeen, Snøhetta involved Scottish artists whose works were combined with those by Norwegian artists Kjell Nupen, Bård Breivik and Kristian Blystad, thus giving visitors the opportunity to get to know the artistic works of the two countries, appreciating similarities and differences. At Maggie's Cardiff, the painting *Self Portrait* by local artist Osi Rhys Osmond, who towards the end of his life decided to donate it to Maggie's, has always been present in the architects' ideas for the centre to become the *zeitgeist* of the building. In this centre, as in all centres, art is not limited to painting but extends to land art as well as sculptures, photographs, watercolours, ceramic or glass objects donated by artists or created by Maggie's visitors.

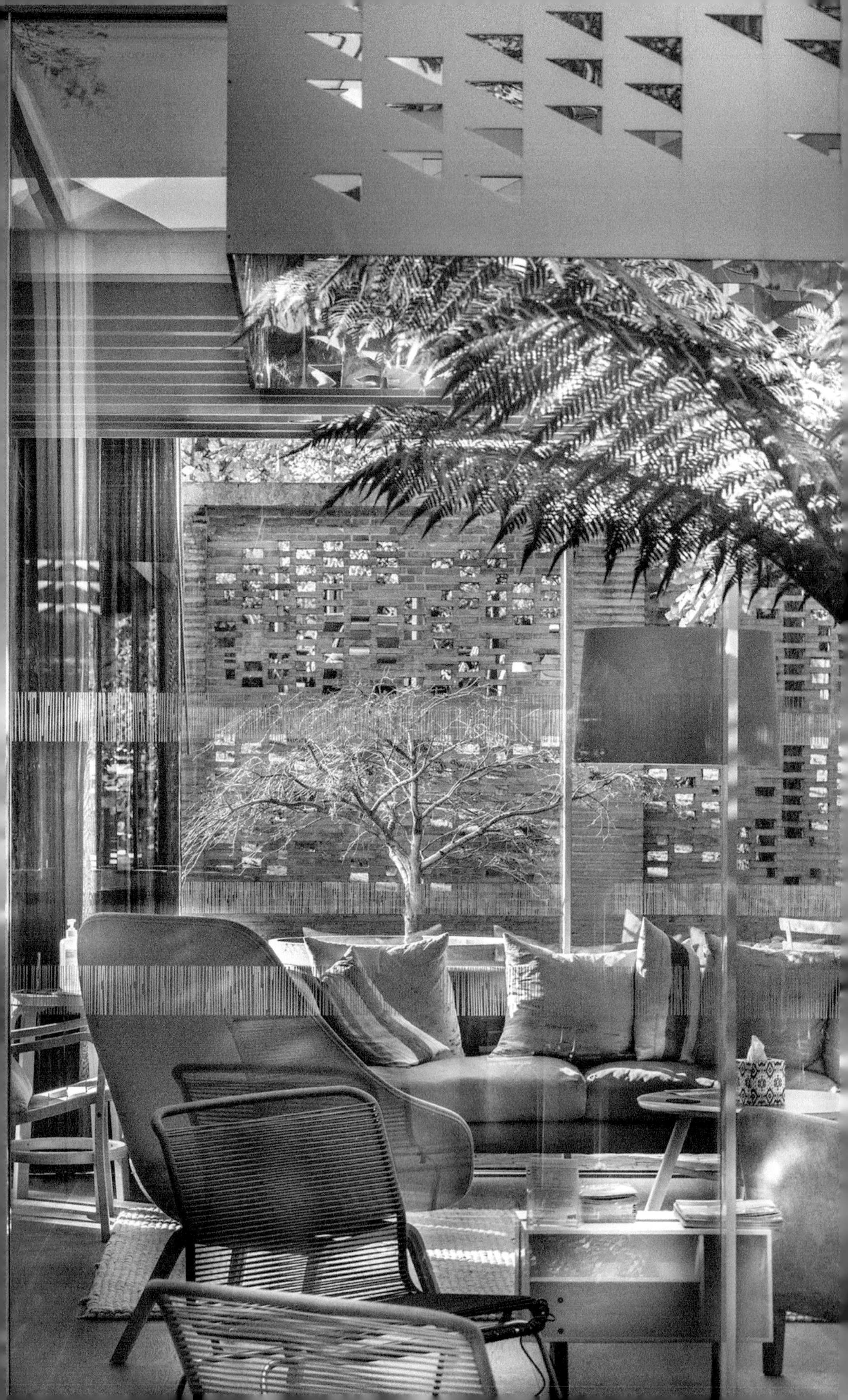

Furniture

The Maggie's centre is designed to feel at home with the types of furniture that we would find in a home: a carpet, a lamp, an old sofa, a fireplace which, combined with cushions, blankets and common objects such as a kettle, a coffee pot, a fruit bowl, create a comfortable and familiar atmosphere. Despite being a contemporary building, but with its "own style and approach versus the modern" (*Jencks, 18.06.2018*), the addition of 'industrial design' pieces, such as a particular lamp or a geometrical coffee table, brings a sophisticated touch. What matters overall is 'comfort' that facilitates new visitors to open up to difficult conversations and those with sleep problems to finally find some peace and be able to fall asleep. Speaking of 'comfort' and how to make people feel at home, Piers Gough describes his Maggie's Nottingham (2011) "traditional with a twist, as it has exaggerated schemes compared to traditional notions of comfort". With chairs and fabrics with a first-modern flavour designed by Paul Smith, the space creates an atmosphere reminiscent of the interiors of Adolf Loos (*Gough, 16.05.2018*).

Compared to a traditional healthcare facility, where furniture usually can't be moved, Maggie's furniture is in constant motion. In particular, chairs—objects of primary importance—move continuously throughout the day. However, for Wendy James (Garber&James), the author of Maggie's Forth Valley (2017) and Maggie's Swansea (2011) on behalf of the late Kisho Kurokawa, even the fixed seats, arranged on the edge of the space, are important because they generate "a sense of order" that transfers calm and tranquillity to the users. Conversely, the scattered chairs bring variety and movement to the space and free the mind of the visitors, even if "there must be an order, a sort of unspoken rule, which makes you understand that things will return to the right place" (*James, 13.06.2018*). At Maggie's Aberdeen (2013), which more than any other centre is called "hug" due to its 'egg-shape' and round space, the *Pelican chairs* envelop those who sit inside, welcoming people with a sense of embrace (*Aabø, 02.11.2018*). As visitors say, the atmosphere that the furnishings, together with the architecture, art and nature create makes people feel cared for, with the same care with which the building is cared for.

Gardens

During my interview with the co–clients, Laura and Marcia, who argued that Maggie's doesn't claim to heal anyone and therefore is not a 'therapeutic environment', it at least emerged that if Maggie's has therapeutic power, that power is in the garden. "I think the only healing way is with the garden" (*Lee, 18.05.2019*). And this is because Laura Lee knows that, beyond the normal mental restoration that comes from nature, Maggie's gardens do much more. As Lily Jencks (2022) explains, the original concept contained in her mother's book *The Chinese Garden* (1978) was that the small Chinese garden represents the miniature of the macrocosm of the world that connects us to something bigger than ourselves. Following the creed of her mother, at Maggie's Glasgow, Lily created a place of meditation

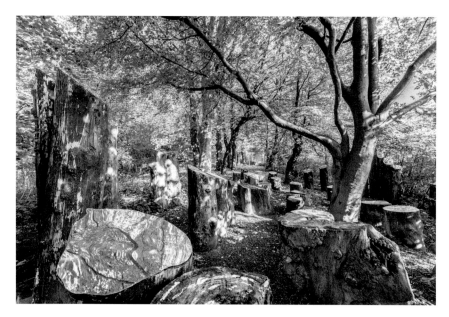

FIGURE 3.17   Maggie's Gardens do much more than ordinary gardens, just like the woodland meditation place designed by Lily Jencks at Maggie's Glasgow (2011) (©Marco Castelli Nirmal).

in the woods by covering the stumps of ancient trees with mirrors that now serve as seats, a small area of peace that makes people feel part of the universe (Figure 3.17).

To generate wellbeing in people, looking at nature is essential. At Maggie's, as the Brief asks, "it is important to be able to look out and even step out from as many of the internal spaces as possible even if it is only into a planted courtyard". When we observe our favourite landscape, as Damasio (1994) explains, the signals coming from the landscape are processed within the brain but also have an impact on the body proper. There is a physiological reason for this. The reason why the body reacts, feeling emotions, when we perceive a landscape—which we do to maintain homeostasis, i.e. the state of functional balance—is that both emotions and homeostasis are regulated in the same place in the brain (brainstem), becoming part of the same biological process (Mallgrave, 2013). As Sternberg (2009) argues, this explains why hotel guests are willing to pay more for a "room with a view".

> Think of viewing a favourite landscape. (…) Signals about the landscape are processed inside the brain. (…) As knowledge pertinent to the landscape is activated internally from dispositional representations in those various brain areas, the rest of the body participates in the process. Sooner or later, the viscera are made to react to the images you are seeing, and to the images your memory is generating internally, relative to what you see. Eventually, when a memory of the seen landscape is formed, that memory will be a neural record of many of the organismic changes just described, some of which happen in the brain itself (the image

constructed for the outside world, together with the images constituted from the memory) and some of which happen in the body proper (…) Perceiving is as much about acting on the environment as it is about receiving signals from it.

(Damasio, 1994, pp. 224–225)

While it is essential to have "a view of nature" (Keswick, 1994) and be connected to the natural environment from within the centre, at Maggie's, it is equally important to enjoy the landscape when arriving at or leaving the centre. Acting as a buffer between the stressful experience lived in the hospital and the reassuring welcome they will receive at Maggie's, or between visiting the centre and returning home, the landscape that visitors pass through offers them a variety of sensory stimuli, from scents that capture their sense of smell, to artistic landscapes that invite movement, to eye-catching sculptures that distract and please. In the garden created by Charles Jencks in collaboration with David Page (Page\Park) for Maggie's Highlands (2002)—a metaphor for living with cancer told through the division of tumour cells—the arrival path is marked by two mounds (representing two single cells), which invite the visitor to climb on them to enjoy the view from above, to contemplate the truth of nature, to meditate on the beauties and struggles of life (Jencks, 2015). Visible from above, the interweaving of the building—an overturned mound—with the landscape—a void—metaphorically represents cell division, i.e.mitosis, reminding visitors that it is possible to live with cancer (Figure 3.18).

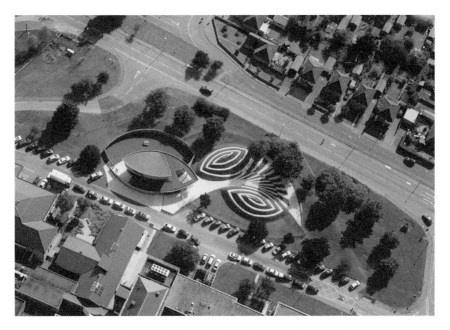

FIGURE 3.18 At Maggie's Highlands (2002) the landscape is a metaphor for living with cancer told through the division of cancer cells (Courtesy of Maggie's).

Among the various forms that Maggie's gardens take is that of the vegetable gardens which requires greater commitment on the part of the organisation and the presence of gardeners; but it is also an opportunity for visitors to contribute and demonstrate reciprocity. At Maggie's Manchester, replacing the staff, this type of landscape plays a different role than the one normally played by nature. Keeping people busy in the care for and harvesting of the land's products to bring them to the centre, vegetable gardens and greenhouses are "a good way to lower the defences and open up to others" (*Haylock, 12.06.2018*) (Figure 3.19).

If in the past the garden was thought of as the final act of the project, with the latest update of the Architectural Brief—which consequently took the name of Architecture and Landscape Brief, 2015—Maggie's has definitively understood how central it is to design the landscape together with the architecture and not afterwards. Considering that no Maggie's centre has ever been designed without a garden, already with the 2007 update of Maggie's Brief, the architectural design was conceived as an integration between building and landscape, which means that, in addition to the architects, Maggie's has since also commissioned landscape architects and made them work together. For example, for Maggie's West London (2008), Dan Pearson worked alongside Ivan Harbour (RSHP), both considering architecture and nature to be of equal weight. Inspired by Maggie Keswick's book (1978), the two designers gave shape to a building—characterised by a high orange wall that wraps around

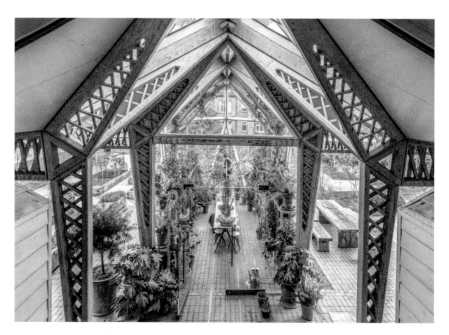

FIGURE 3.19 Maggie's uses the greenhouse to keep people busy taking care of the land's products, a good way to lower defenses and open up to others (Maggie's Manchester, 2016) (©Marco Castelli Nirmal).

itself like a "nautilus"—that makes room for many courtyards that resemble those of a Chinese house. As Marcia Blackenham commented (*18.05.2019*), being able to see something green from every corner of the building makes Maggie's West London (2008) seem a world so far away from the nearby gigantic hospital of Charing Cross and London bus traffic.

Charles Jencks' Legacy: Icons, Metaphors, Hybrid and Placebo Effect

Charles Jencks described Maggie's centres as 'mini-icons' containing 'multiple metaphors'.

> They all imply various metaphors that connect us with nature, some even with cosmos, but they also allow for different readings. They all give presence to the basic questions of 'living well, suffering and dying'.
>
> (Jencks, 2012, p. 37)

As he explains, in the past the iconic was that of the monument based on symbols that people knew well, such as the shape of the temple and the Christian cross. Today the iconic building is much more striking than individual symbols. When we are faced with cancer, in a continuous oscillation between preparing to die and the struggle for life, the unconscious solution is, like in the past, to orient ourselves to nature.

> 'Take your pain to the cosmos' is a Christian *nostrum* dating back to prehistoric times; only nature is large enough to contain it.
>
> (Jencks, 2017, p. 69)

Since only nature is large enough to contain pain, the 'Christian horizon' is a natural metaphor for 'hope' which, in healthcare architecture, is essential to convey the idea that there is still a future (Jencks, 2014). This is why all of Maggie's centres offer infinite views of the horizon and, at the same time, small contained nooks looking towards tiny gardens or the sky (Figures 3.20 and 3.21). It is to the complex, multiple and contradictory human emotions that arise in illness that the minimalist and sober or highly expressive 'architecture of hope' of the different Maggie's centres can respond. The context of the hospital grounds is usually dark and melancholy. By contrast, the Maggie's centre has a 'cheerful' and non-institutional feel. The reason behind the 'iconicity' of some of the buildings finds its answer here. Yet, others are very quiet, almost "hidden in the forest". An ideal and utopian project, as Charles Jencks considers it (Jencks, 2019), the Maggie's centre combines four different types of buildings and their opposites in one.

> We are 'homely', but we are not a home; we are religious, but we are not a church; we love art, but we are not a museum; we help patients, but we are not a hospital. The work is essentially gripping.
>
> (Jencks, 18.06.2018)

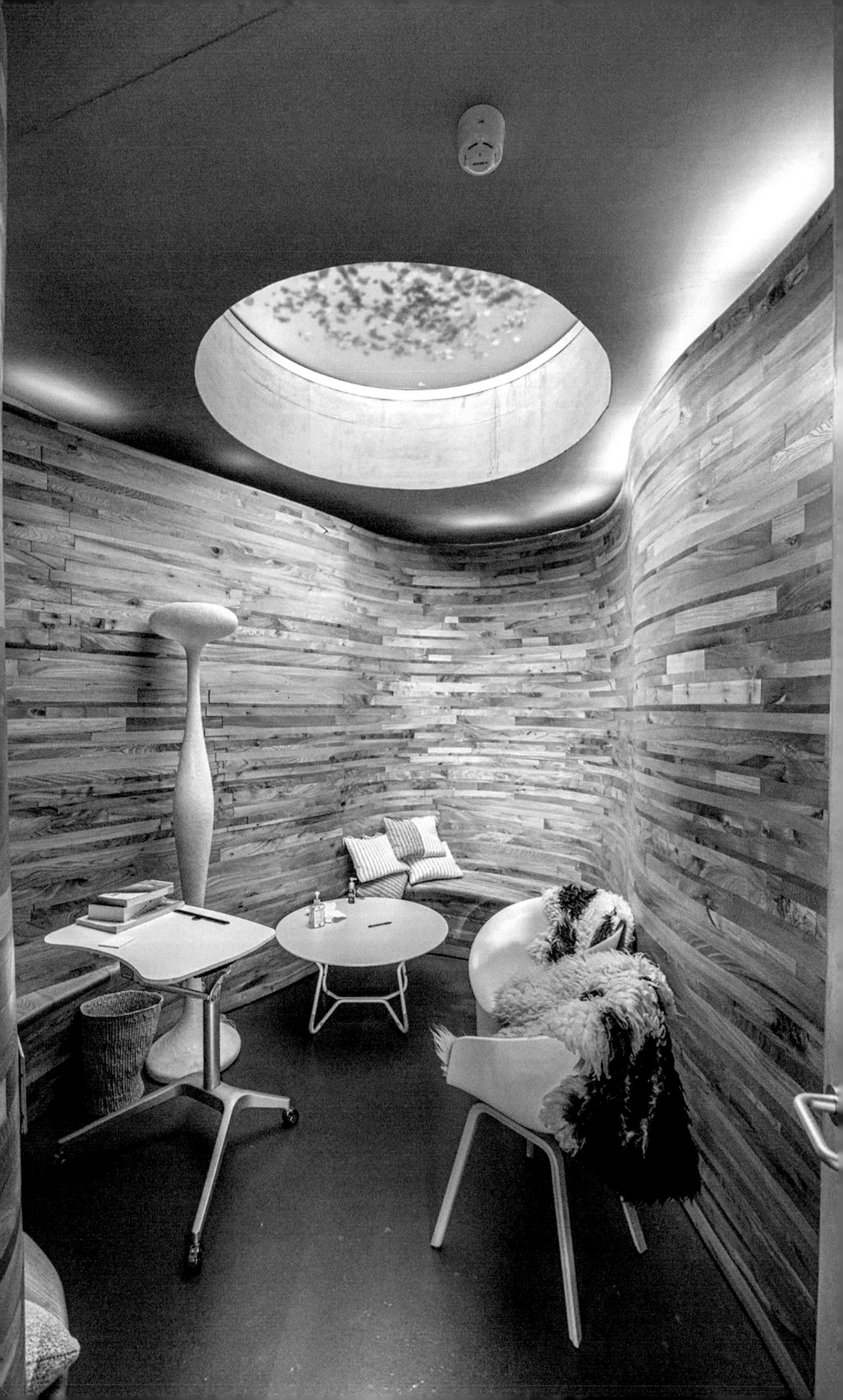

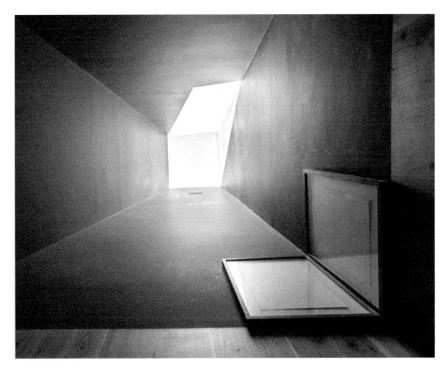

FIGURES 3.20–3.21   All Maggie centres offer endless views of the horizon or narrow views through small cozy nooks, over tiny gardens or up to the sky (Maggie's Glasgow, 2011) (©Marco Castelli Nirmal), (Maggie's Cardiff, 2019) (©Anthony Coleman).

Informal as a home, the Maggie's centre is designed to be cosy, domestic, small in size for socialising, sharing experiences at the kitchen table or while making a coffee or tea at the counter, to learn relaxation and how to eat well. At the same time it is also a place of art, where you can take art therapy courses and enjoy the works of art that entertain and distract. Furthermore, it is a place of healing where the motto 'empower the patient' philosophy combined with information on cancer care helps to manage one's disease and, finally, it is a spiritual place where people, grappling with some last questions, can find the necessary intimacy in secluded corners even within large common areas. Jencks had theorised the hybrid since 1985, even stating that it was hard to get.

> The hybrid is difficult to achieve, certainly more demanding than single-minded attention to aesthetics and technology that the brilliant Mies van der Rohe followed. It is also as a language richer in scope, making full use of the architectural means including ornament, symbolism, craftsmanship, polychromies and metaphor.
>
> (Jencks, 1985, p. 8)

Another attribute that Charles Jencks assigns to the Maggie's Centre is that of the 'placebo effect'. Its discovery was marked by the famous quote by the American philosopher William James.

> The greatest revolution in our generation is the discovery that human beings, by changing the inner attitudes of their minds, can change the outer aspects of their lives.
>
> (James, 1890, quoted in Jencks, 2012, p. 31)

As is well known, a placebo is a 'fake' cure that works because it acts on the patients' belief. Since the 1950s and especially after the publication of the work of Henry K. Beecher (1955), the scientific community has taken placebo results seriously, as placebos have been shown to work well as conventional medications in some cases, especially those dealing with psychogenic problems (Jencks, 2012). Consequently, Charles wondered:

> How can phoney things work? [And, moving the discussion to Architecture] How do we gauge the effect of a building on health if, like the placebo effect, it is partly in the mind? Or, is there an architectural placebo?
>
> (Jencks, 2012, p. 31)

Because in the placebo effect, blue pills work statistically better than red ones, especially for diligent patients (Moerman, 2002), translated into architectural language, Jencks argued that "style does not matter if patients who go to Maggie's diligently may do better than those who do not" (Jencks, 2012, p. 33). Charles explained to me that in the case of the Maggie's centre, this fact is amplified by the quality of the building, the style and, above all, by the feelings and activity offered by the staff. However, not wanting to give too much weight to the question "Can architecture affect health?", Jencks has always maintained that Maggie's architecture and the arts have an indirect effect on people with cancer, because they first pass through the staff. "The architecture supports the staff which in turn supports the patients" (Jencks, 2012, p. 37).

In an effort to keep alive the attributes that Charles Jencks assigned to the Maggie's centre and that may be lost now that he is gone, while reinforcing his idea that architecture and health are closely linked, this book aims to take one step further in demonstrating that the beneficial effects experienced by the visitor come directly from the building without going through the staff. However, since what Maggie's does is to convey to people with cancer the message that 'suffering' is a normal part of life and, as such, it is better to accept it, and since therapeutic architecture has no rules, but rather as Jencks argued, "only the strength of its spirit, the harshness of its challenge and the sense of provocation", to generate these effects, once suffering is accepted, then we must believe that architecture comes to our rescue. This is confirmed by the history of humanity, which has always believed in the act of building monuments and symbols using architecture as a placebo to overcome great adversities.

> Architecture gives a perspective, a message of hope, at least in a religious or faith context: monuments, sanctuaries and temples that man built in the history to celebrate or thank divinities after survival through epidemic times witness the deep connection between architecture, religion and health. The ritual monumental setting, from Stonehenge (3000–2000 B.C.) to the Lourdes Sanctuary (1858)—in a way, early examples of architectural placebo—constitute the spiritual landscape of healing environments.
>
> (Jencks, 2012, p. 37)

References

BBC (2016) 'Building Hope: The Maggie's Centres', Full BBC Documentary. https://www.youtube.com/watch?v=QkVcZuAikrI&t=2083s&ab_channel=nomadwariror

Beecher, H. K. (1955) 'The Powerful Placebo', *Journal of the American Medical Association*, 159(17), pp. 1602–1606

Berthoz, A. (2000) *The Brain's Sense of Movement*. Boston, MA: Harvard University Press

Brennan, S. (2015) 'Patterns of Neurons Firing'. Interview with Sabina Brennan. Interviewed by N. McLaughlin and Y. Manolopoulou for Losing Myself. http://www.losing-myself.ie/pages/patterns-neurons-firing/

Damasio, A. (1994) *Descartes' Error: Emotion, Reason, and the Human Brain*. London: Vintage

Darwin, C. (1874) *The Descendent of Man, and Selection in Relation to Sex*. London: John Murray

Eberhard, J. P. (2009) 'Applying Neuroscience to Architecture', *Neuroview*, 62(6), pp. 753–756

Erwine, B. (2016) *Creating Sensory Spaces: The Architecture of the Invisible*. New York: Routledge

Frisone, C. (2021) *The Role of Architecture in the Therapeutic Environment. The Case of the Maggie's Cancer Care Centre*, Doctoral Thesis, Faculty of Technology, Design and Environment, Oxford Brookes University. https://doi.org/10.24384/0ejy-7815

Howells, L. (2016) 'Synergy between People and Place', TEDxTalks. https://www.youtube.com/watch?v=tvE78D30CbQ

Jencks, C. (1985) *Modern Movements in Architecture*. London: Penguin Group

Jencks, C. (2012) *Can Architecture Affect Your Health*. London: ArtEZ Press

Jencks, C. (2014). 'Charles Jencks: Can Architecture Affect Your Health?'. New York School of Interior Design, 6 March. https://www.youtube.com/watch?v=QcjYEzD9jSs&ab_channel=NewYorkSchoolofInteriorDesign

Jencks, C. (2015) *The Architecture of Hope: Maggie's Cancer Caring Centres* (2nd ed.). London: Frances Lincoln

Jencks, C. (2017) 'Maggie's Architecture: The Deep Affinities between Architecture and Health', *Architectural Design*, 87(2), pp. 66–75

Jencks, C. (2019). Architecture of Maggie's: Charles Jencks with Alex de Rijke and Benedetta Tagliabue. Building Centre, London, 29 May. https://www.youtube.com/watch?v=BK3N-1bBwGc&ab_channel=BuildingCentre

Jencks, L. (2022) 'Maggie's Cancer Centre Gardens: Herbs, Habitat and a Search for Deep Meaning', in Frisone, C. (ed.) *Maggie's Centres: On the Road*. Florence: Forma Edizioni, pp. 19–22

Keswick, M. (1978) *The Chinese Garden: History, Art & Architecture*. New York: John Wiley & Sons

Keswick, M. (1994) 'A View from the Frontline'. Revised and reprinted in 2003 and 2007. https://maggies-staging.s3.amazonaws.com/media/filer_public/5b/f6/5bf6f8c7-37e4-4b0a-b09d-6ad48d66387d/view-from-the-front-line.pdf

Losing Myself (2016) Losing Myself, Biennale Architettura Venice. https://www.niallmclaughlin.com/projects/losing-myself-biennale-venice/

Maggie's Brief (2015) 'Architecture and Landcape Brief'. https://maggies-staging.s3 .amazonaws.com/media/filer_public/e0/3e/e03e8b60-ecc7-4ec7-95a1-18d9f9c4e7c9/ maggies_architecturalbrief_2015.pdf

Maggie's Professionals (2023) [Information] For Healthcare Professionals. https://www. maggies.org/about-us/healthcare-professionals/

Maggie's Videos (2019) 'Breathing Space'. https://www.youtube.com/watch?v=j8EhZJucHwc

Mallgrave, H. F. (2013) *Architecture and Embodiment: The implications of the New Sciences and Humanities for Design*. London and New York: Routledge

Moerman, D. (2002) *Meaning, Medicine and the 'Placebo effect'*. Cambridge: Cambridge University Press

Sternberg, E. (2009) *Healing Spaces: The Science of Place and Wellbeing*. Cambridge, MA: Belknap Press of Harvard University Press

Van der Kolk, B. (2015) *The Body Keeps the Score: Mind, Brain and Body in the Transformation of Trauma*. London: Penguin

4

MAGGIE'S FUNDAMENTALS

Maggie's 'Therapeutikós'

As seen in the introduction, the difference between 'therapeutic' and 'healing' does not lie so much in their current meaning (usually the former refers to a psychological benefit and the latter mainly to a physical/medical one), but in the etymology of the word which reveals the subject of reference: generally, it is the therapist who offers the therapies and the patient who needs healing. Once this difference did not exist, since 'mind' and 'body' were treated holistically and *therapeutes* (Θεραπευτές) and *invalids* lived together, the ones offering therapies and being with the others who, thanks to this coexistence, found healing in suffering. This is what characterised Asclepian Healing, the medicine practiced by the mythological god Asclepius, whose emblem of a rod with a coiled serpent is still today the symbol that represents the need for attention required in medicine (Eldestein, 1945, cited in Kearney, 2009).

Asclepian Healing was divided into three stages: the stage of purification, that of preparation and that of true healing practiced by Asclepius. After walking a long way to reach the sanctuary and obtain healing, the sick were welcomed by the priests (*therapeutes*) and their assistants who organised "practices and rituals at the temple" (2009, p. 41). While family members were housed in the *katagòghion*, the sick were purified through fasting, bathing in the local mineral springs, and rituals that stimulated emotions through artistic and recreational activities (Kerenyi, 1959, cited in Kearney, 2009). Once the preparation phase was completed, the sick entered the *abaton*—the sacred dormitory near the temple accessible only to them—where Asclepius would later heal them by incubation. In the "darkness of the night", while the sick were "sleeping on the ground" and "non-poisonous snakes crawled freely between their bodies", Asclepius would appear in their sleep to practice the healing, which was connected to "the deep aspects of the psyche

DOI: 10.4324/9781003244516-4

rather than in the luminous consciousness of the surface mind" (Kearney, 2009, p. 44). Upon awakening, the sick person, who had dreamed of being healed by the god, had to leave a thank-you contribution and remember the dream, because it was in the phenomenological experience of the dream that healing took place (Suárez De La Torre, 2005). So, not the subsequent interpretation of the dream, but the dream itself was healing. "The healing was in the encounter with the dream as epiphany. The healing was the dreaming" (Kearney, 2009, p. 45).

The preparatory phase preceding healing could last for days, and in the meantime the sick lived the life at the centre. As a prerequisite for meeting the god Asclepius, patients had to reach a flexible state of mind that would allow them to accept suffering, made tolerable by the "compassionate and caring attitude of those who care for them and stay with them in suffering" (Kearney, 2009, p. xxii), supported by an "articulated environment" which was a significant factor for health.

By introducing the theme of suffering here, I want to sensitise the reader to the fact that, in neurobiology, suffering is considered necessary for living beings because it increases their attention to pain signals and prompts them to act to avert the worst, ensuring their survival. According to Damasio (2000), in fact, subjects born with a bizarre condition known as the 'congenital absence of pain' do not acquire normal behavioural strategies. Indeed, pain is a lever to react instinctively and develop correlated decision-making strategies (Damasio, 1994). In this, knowing the biology of emotions and feelings that relates to suffering helps to understand the causes and reduce human discomfort (Damasio, 2004).

Having discovered the affinities between the *therapeutikós* of Asclepian Healing, based on the participation of the *therapeutes* in the healing of the sick supported by a magnificent landscape, and the psychological support offered by Maggie's, based on the caring attitude of the staff towards the visitors sustained by an uplifting architecture, is what prompted me to elect this compassionate attitude as Maggie's first fundamental, naming it Maggie's *therapeutikós*. Evidence of this resemblance is contained in Kearney's narration of the story of Leto, a 50-year-old sick woman, from southern Crete, who had walked to the temple of Asclepius in Lissos to have her right breast, now in an advanced state of disease, healed.

Welcomed by Cleo, with whom she would go through the stages of purification and preparation, on the day of the incubation Leto was ready to go up to the temple with Cleo and, together with other incubants, before meeting Asclepius, perform a dance made of harmonious movements in pleasant spaces. To achieve flexibility or "the right frame of mind to undergo the process of incubation" (Meier, 1989, quoted in Kearney, 2009, p. 44), *therapeutes* and *invalids* were together in suffering creating a synergistic collaboration, a 'fluid dance'.

By now it was dark and others were making their way up the road to the temple. Cleo walked beside Leto. Soon they came to an opening among the olive trees, not far from the temple, where they joined with other incubants and the priests and priestesses in a circle around a blazing fire. Together they all joined in an invocation to the god.

(Kearney, 2009, p. 94)

In addition to offering therapeutic effects, the peculiarity of a therapeutic environment is, in fact, that of inviting everyone to attend and participate (from *therapeuein* 'to attend, treat' and from *theraps* 'attendant') and to get involved, together, through a remarkable stimulation of the senses. "Asclepian healing depends on both patients and carers using the 'inner senses' of emotion, instinct, intuition, and somatic awareness" (2009, p. 46) to be found "in the subjective experience of inner transformation and healing of patients" (Kearney, 2009, p. xxii).

Just like with Asclepian healing practice, where patients were left alone because it is in personal struggle that they found harmony, balance, and personal development (Kearney, 2009), Maggie's support programme promotes the experience of individual meditation on the choices that are offered. Indeed, Maggie's programme tells its visitor that it is a difficult road to walk alone, but that 'you are not alone', in a way that is strikingly similar to how Kearney describes it:

She felt a wave of grief ascending like a spring and tears began to flow. For what seemed like ages she wept (…) Leto knew that she was both alone and not alone.

(Kearney, 2009, p. 95)

At the same time, to make them *feel included,* Maggie's staff constantly assist the visitors, "because it is impossible to help patients in difficulty without entering into the experience with them" (Kearney, 2009, p. 46). Moreover*,* within the philosophy of 'kitchenism', according to which "the centrality of food and drink allows people to enter and exit without declaring themselves, trying things, listening or going out unnoticed" (Jencks and Heathcote, 2010, p. 13), at Maggie's, visitors *feel at home.* Finally, as seen in the previous chapter, before she died, Maggie Keswick won her last battle with cancer, leaving behind a fundamental aspect of her programme: the paradox of the liberating therapy of struggle and humour, which we also find in Asclepian healing.

By now Leto was feeling more at home. She found it difficult to understand how a place like this could have such an atmosphere of peace, hope and even humour.

(Kearney, 2009, p. 91)

Finally, again as described by Kerneay about Asclepian Healing, which is "a process whereby one who is limited in his or her ability to help stays with another in suffering in a way that allows healing to happen" (Kearney, 2009, p. 47), the Maggie's centre, open and free, tells its users that "architecture provides a unique way of helping people relate to each other" (*Lee, 16.10.2019*). And in making them *feel valued,* Maggie's tells them that, in suffering, "we're not the only ones" (Howells, 2016, 8:53).

> It also allowed her to meet and talk with others who, like her, had come to the shrine in search of healing. She heard many stories of suffering and healing. Just as the waters cleansed her body, these stories bathed her soul.
>
> (Kearney, 2009, p. 91)

Analysing Kearney's story and drawing a parallel with Maggie's reality, we essentially learn two things: the first, that in a therapeutic environment the spatial and social experience that activates all the emotions and feelings seen above is often accompanied by an incomprehensible feeling ("I can't explain it"). In fact, even Leto, finally says:

> It wasn't really like a dream; it seems like it really happened. It's strange… I'm the same 'me' as yesterday and yet… something is different. (…) I can't explain it.
>
> (Kearney, 2009, p. 100)

The second is that since ancient times the basic human needs of the individual have always been the same: *to feel included, to feel at home, to feel valued.* These requirements or principles, which emphasise the human value of dignity as fundamental to the Architecture of Care, are intrinsic in the Maggie's centre through both the architecture and the support programme; in particular the principle of *inclusion*—which is usually absent in healthcare—is primary in counteracting solitude and depersonalisation.

In the same interview held by Níall McLaughlin and Yeoryia Manolopoulou as part of the research on dementia (2016) seen in the previous chapter—where Sabrina Brennan (2015) explains that the 'staff station' creates segregation and therefore the opposite of *inclusion*—it emerges that the need *to feel at home* develops widely in healthcare environments, especially in institutions for the elderly where people are forced to live in places they no longer recognise as 'home' and which they don't feel they belong to. Since memories are integrated with behaviours, feeling disoriented, the elderly will always look for familiar spaces from the past in the current space and, in an attempt to adjust to the new situation, they will often talk about their upstairs bedroom even though the building is only one storey. Also, not *feeling valued* creates a state of anxiety. Studies conducted in Neuroethics show that unfairness or lack of recognition of merit causes sadness to the point that even monkeys, when they experience this feeling, no longer collaborate (*Pallanti, 07.10.2022*). The danger of sadness and anxiety—which are a "state dependent on processing in the brain"—is that they cause a decline in the immune system which leads the body to be susceptible to infections and, as a direct or otherwise consequence, to develop some types of cancer. As Damasio says: "One can die of a broken heart" (1994, p. 120).

Constituting the first fundamental, Maggie's *therapeutikós* is inherent in the architecture and Maggie's programme. By making people feel like individuals, Maggie's openness helps visitors *feel included*. Pretty quickly, Maggie's familiarity—or 'kitchenism'—puts people with cancer at ease and they begin to *feel at home*. Over time, Maggie's unconventionality, that which makes people aware, helps visitors *feel valued*. Inviting users (staff, doctors, people with cancer, family, friends) to participate and share, just like Leto, "many stories of suffering and healing" (Kearny, 2009, p. 91), Maggie's *therapeutikós* is the key to creating a synergistic collaboration, a metaphorical 'fluid dance' of people in synergy with the place, enabling a mental flexibility that allows them to tolerate what was previously intolerable.

The Architectural Brief

Maggie's second fundamental resides in the Architectural Brief (2015) upon which the Maggie's centre is designed and managed. The reason why I proposed to elect it as such lies in its strength of extraordinary resemblance to that of the Benedictine *Rule* (547 A.D.), the brief on which the Monastery of Montecassino (Italy) was founded by Saint Benedict of Nursia in 530 A.D. Akin to the ancient chart that is a concentration of the architecture, programme and life values of the monastery, Maggie's Brief governs the architects' project, informs life at the centre, and embodies Maggie's mission. Furthermore, just like the *Rule*, the Architectural Brief requires an architecture aimed at supporting its users in carrying out their work while finding safety and comfort. Although in 2015, as mentioned in the previous chapter, it was renamed "Maggie's Architecture and Landscape Brief" to promote integrated architecture-nature design, in this book I will refer to it simply as 'Architectural Brief' or 'Maggie's Brief'.

An architectural brief is a written statement of a client's needs, on the basis of which an architect is called to respond with a design conforming to the original request (Salisbury, 1998). Born in the 1950s in Great Britain to regulate public sector buildings (houses, hospitals and schools), the brief was theorised for the first time in the 1970s in the United States, where architects less convinced of the "form-follows-function" design strategy questioned the principles accepted until then. Carrying forward the idea of "learning from practice to write a brief", for example, Louis Kahn (1901–1974) was adamant that a real brief could only be written once the building was built (Blyth and Worthington, 2007). A great contribution to the definition of the brief and its use in architecture came from Christopher Alexander who, with his book *A Pattern Language* (Alexander, Ishikawa and Silverstein, 1977), helped identify the structures of the architectural lexicon. Describing a scientifically organised system through 253 models aimed at solving common problems in cities, the book served as an architectural brief for many architects of later generations, including Maggie's first architect, Richard Murphy, whose Maggie's Edinburgh (1996), in line with Kahn's suggestion, served to write Maggie's Brief. For architects it is indeed true that, as Ivan Harbour (RSHP) states, "Design only finishes when buildings are built" (*20.07.2018*).

In addition to providing a physical description, a brief can also define how users will use the future building. Throughout history, examples of briefs that suggest the social, religious or philosophical mission of the building range from the pontifical *brevis*—documents with the meaning of "letter, short communication, summary", containing instructions in a more synthetic and less solemn form than a *bulla* (Santacroce, 2015)—to the already seen *Rule* of St. Benedict of Nursia (480–547 A.D.), up to most recent regulations of educational philosophies such as those of Rudolf Steiner (1861–1925) or Maria Montessori (1870–1952). Among these and various other precedents, in my investigation, the Benedictine *Rule* turned out to be the most significant reference to the Maggie's centre, also for its human contents and tacit organisation.

The Benedictine *Rule* or *Sancta Regula* is the 'brief' written by St. Benedict between 530 and 547A.D., following the foundation of the Monastery of Montecassino in 530 A.D. Direct and concise, this seemingly modest and simple booklet has for centuries been the source of inspiration for royal rulers, from Charlemagne (VIII A.D.) to the French dominators (XVII–XVIII A.D.). Feeling the need for a 'more orderly organisation', over time many have appealed to the *Rule* which has proven to be unique for practicality and flexibility. Inexhaustible in principles, values and citations, never out of time, still today it continues to represent an example of perfect organisation that is easily applicable to a modern company (Folador, 2006).

> For 1500 years, Benedictine monasteries have been an illuminating example of what it means to live and work in a context where everyone has clear goals and objectives, roles and tasks and knows how to make the community their strength. A perfect organisation that has spanned the centuries and that can say many things to the managerial world, thanks to the correct management of shared values, widespread leadership and the ability to make people work together who are motivated and aware of their responsibilities.
>
> (Folador, 2006*, back cover)

The construction of Montecassino saw St. Benedict engaged as an architect, organiser and inspirer of the new monastery and its community of monks—equally skilled architects and builders—until his death in 547 A.D. In describing how the community life was to be conducted, the rigour and the objectives to be achieved, always looking ahead and trying to work as a team, the *Rule* addresses individual monks with a clear structure and a pragmatic message. Composed of 73 short chapters, the document invites the monks to create a building whose architecture is "great and powerful" and "that everyone should feel his own", capable of reflecting the strength of the community. At the same time, St. Benedict calls the monks to their daily work, showing concern for their personal problems, aware of the fact that everyone, even the one with the humblest task, is an individual, a valid component of the community who contributes in a personal and decisive way (Folador, 2006). In Benedictine culture, in fact, in addition to the religious one, also the lay side linked to the uniqueness of the person plays a fundamental role (Folador, 2006).

Both founded on 'spiritual' and 'concrete' pillars, finding their strength in an organised life and shared values, the *Rule* and the Monastery of Montecassino constitute a single work, which Benedict knew would never die because it was entrusted not so much to the stones of a building, but to a small booklet which, even before being multiplied into parchments, was preserved in the memory and heart of people (Salvatorelli, 1983). This concept is now replicated in the Maggie's centre and a new Rule, the Architectural Brief.

Maggie's Architectural Brief derives from the *Blueprint for a Cancer Caring Centre* the text that Maggie was trying to write before her death in 1995. The Blueprint itself originated from *A View from the Front Line* (1994) further developed in *Empowering the Patient* (1994), the text that urged patients to self-sufficiency and moved the idea of simply transforming a room at the end of the corridor of the Edinburgh hospital into that of creating "a welcoming place near the hospital, with an office and a library" (Blakenham, 2007, p. 3).

> Each person visiting the centre would be helped to find his or her own best way of coping with the disease. There was to be no 'right way'. The centre was to be a haven, where the range of use would extend from a cup of tea you could make yourself in a friendly kitchen to attending weekly support groups led by a clinical psychologist.
>
> (Blakenham, 2007, p. 4)

The idea of the original 'CCC Cancer Care Centre' and writing a brief developed strongly only after Laura Lee went to the United States in 1994 to explore Californian hospices with Maggie. As Charles told me:

> When Laura Lee came to visit us in Los Angeles it was a really important moment; it was when Laura, Maggie, Mike Dixon and Bob Leonard and others formed a team. It took 2 years to write it.
>
> (*Jencks, 27.04.2018*)

As mentioned in the previous chapter, the Architectural Brief was written by Charles, Laura and Marcia in 1998 and was only two pages long. The brief was revised with minor changes in 2003 and, then again, in 2007 to coincide with the reissue of *A View from the Front Line* (Keswick, 1994), which now included the 'Foreword' and the chapter 'Maggie's centres: Marching On' by Marcia Blakenham. Also supported by this publication, while retaining its brevity and apparent simplicity, in less than 10 years, the Brief had clearly become more challenging.

> Maggie's asks a lot of its buildings and hence of its architects. We expect the physical space to do a significant amount of our work for us.
>
> (Architectural Brief, 2007, p. 1)

The current Architectural Brief (2015), still concise and vague, has remained essentially unchanged since then. While not very specific in terms of functional space requirements, it well describes what people must feel when using the building. It start by saying:

> Please be patient with us if this seems like a long preamble to the specific spatial requirements of a Maggie's Centre. More than anything else this brief is about the feelings we need the design of these places to convey to the people who will be visiting them.
>
> (Maggie's Brief, 2015, p. 2)

In reading it, seemingly very simple and not difficult to answer, Piers Gough gave a perfect interpretation.

> It's very British, you have to read between the lines. It is not obvious what they are asking you. Just the idea that they challenge you on what you can do for them stimulates your imagination.
>
> (*Gough, 16.05.2018*)

This white space "between the lines" constitutes the portion of freedom left to the architects in designing their own centre converging in it a great deal of wisdom and knowledge that will help generate the feelings required by the Architectural Brief. The result is a personal interpretation that makes each centre a unique exemplar, different from all the other buildings, but which, in line with the Brief, communicates the same stimulating effects as all the others. The idea that the architecture should be stimulating is confirmed by the Brief itself.

> (…) these little buildings should not pat you on the head, patronise you by being too cosy. They should rise to the occasion, just as you, the person needing help, is having to rise to the occasion of one of the most difficult challenges any of us is likely to have to face.
>
> (Appendix I, p. 1)

As explained, Maggie's Edinburgh (1996) represents the founding moment of Maggie's project and embodies the quintessence of the Architectural Brief, establishing the cardinal principles of an unprecedented archetype. By placing the open kitchen near the front door and merging it with the open staircase, banishing corridors altogether, Murphy's design created a spatial typology that would later become one of the central concepts of the Architectural Brief. Adopted in all future Maggie's centres, the open-plan model in constant contact with nature is the genesis of the 'spatial interaction rather than walls' principle. As Murphy says:

> The important thing is, as you come in, you can look up and you basically see all the destinations that you might want to go to. So, there's nothing hidden in any way. I always think it's absolutely important, when you go into a building,

if it's possible, that you grasp the geography of the building straightaway; and then people's anxiety level drops down.

(BBC, 2016, 17:05)

Murphy's design, which is not only open but also flexible, has influenced every architect who succeeded him. Recognising that space must adapt to the different needs of people, Maggie's architects design the space to be adaptable to continuous change. As Ellen van Loon (OMA) states, in fact, not being able to predict how people feel, especially when they have a serious illness, architects will have to provide a 'menu' of spaces available to everyone, a 'shell' that allows people to experience a series of emotions depending on the moment (*van Loon, 05.15.2018*).

Instrumental in guiding architects to design an open and flexible building, where architecture, life at the centre and community values coincide, the equally open and flexible Architectural Brief proves to be the cornerstone of Maggie's organisation. With reference to the *Rule* of Saint Benedict (547 A.D.) which, with its clear and pragmatic message, has been the beacon of the greatest rulers for centuries and still represents a model of 'perfect organisation' today, Maggie's Brief will often emerge in this book; in particular, in Chapter 7, the idea of replicating Maggie's archetype, becoming a paradigm, would not be possible without the strength of the Architectural Brief, which lies in its invariability. "What will not vary is the requirement to build a beautiful, small, humane building, which raises your spirits when you walk into it" (Maggie's Brief, 2015, p. 9). Like the monastery which, thanks to the Rule, has proliferated throughout Europe, reaching—including abbeys and convents—an unpredictable number of 75,000 in about 1,500 years (Folador, 2006), the Maggie's centre, to a lesser extent, in just over 25 years, has already multiplied many times and is in a continuous process of growth.

Maggie's Triad and its 'Superb' Product

There are twenty-two [*thirty, today*] centres up and running, six more on the horizon mostly in Britain, and architects have played a major role in their success (…). What I've found surprising, and gratifying, is that most of these centres work very well and architecturally they are 'superb'. There must be several reasons for this, but among them is the challenge of the building task itself. Living with cancer, succumbing to it, fighting and laughing it off, seems to motivate architects to outperform themselves.

(Jencks, 2018, para. 2)

Maggie's third fundamental lies in its Triad, the triangular relationship that is established between the co-clients, the architect and the centre users, governed by the Architectural Brief, when a new building is born. The reason for this choice came from the fact that the project for a Maggie's centre seems to push architects to go beyond themselves, creating a product that, as Charles Jencks defined it, is architecturally "superb".

The triad concept is one of the fundamental characteristics of the architectural system and is the basis of the 'Commissioning of Architecture' process, otherwise known as *Design Brief Management and Procurement* (Masterman, 1992). In architecture, in addition to identifying the document, the term 'brief' also indicates the process through which the client communicates his/her ideas to the architect on the basis of a brief or programme, in order to make efforts that converge towards the common goal represented by the user (Blyth and Worthington, 2007). This triple system involves a close collaboration between the three parties; the lack of a systematic approach to this collaboration is the main obstacle to the success of the project (Yu et al., 2007). This misstep occurs when, for example, the link between the client and the architect becomes too close, while that with the users is minimal or neglected, highlighting an imbalance in the system. Although research on improving briefing practices has shown that clients are the main providers of information (Barrett and Stanley, 1999), users can also be considered a valuable source of knowledge about specific requirements that clients often struggle to capture. Therefore, involving users in the design should improve the efficiency of the briefing process and the value of the *design team* (Zwemmer and den Otter, 2008).

In Maggie's case, co-clients collaborate closely with the architects based on the Architectural Brief; in return, with their architecture, architects respond, on the one hand, to the co-clients and, on the other, to the users. Users (visitors and staff), for their part, are influenced by both the architect and co-clients through the architecture and the support programme, which, together, collaborate on Maggie's mission. Although they constitute the main objective of the project as recipients of the final product of the Triad (the building), following the principle of Zwemmer and den Otter (2008), within the Triad, Maggie's users do not have much weight in the design process, if not through the co-clients who advocate for them.

Yet, the informal conversations I had with the numerous users of the various Maggie's centres have revealed a high level of satisfaction, which in the architectural system is the tip of the balance, what establishes the success of the building (Blyth and Worthington, 2007). It should also be said that, although users have not been actively involved in the design, especially in the past, over time the bond between the architect and the user has strengthened and circumstances have helped. For example, when architects visit existing centres and meet users during the design phase, they collect a lot of information from them, even if it is still not enough to say that users are involved in the design process. By assigning the users an active role within the *design team* of Maggie's Triad, which consists in telling other users about their positive user experience and how to recognise a therapeutic environment, as we will see in Chapter 7, this book intends to encourage all users to become 'user-experts', free to have their say and report it to the architects, ultimately triggering the process that will improve the built environment.

As the title of Salisbury's book *Briefing Your Architect* (1998) suggests, the primary responsibility still remains with the client. In addressing the lesson on the 'not-so-simple' art of communicating the client's needs to the designer to obtain the desired product, Salisbury implies that the architect's competence does not in itself guarantee the result. Furthermore, by using the adjective 'your', Salisbury alludes to a certain dependence of the latter on the former (Fontana, 2007). It is true that history shows that the architect cannot achieve anything [great] without an [inspired] client (De Carlo, 2004, cited in Fontana, 2007). There are many examples of well-known architects whose quality of work has been significantly determined by their clients. Just to name one, while designing the Willey House (1934), even Frank Lloyd Wright was challenged by his client. Modern, courageous, intelligent, curious and a generation younger than Wright, Nancy Willey forced her architect to set aside his initial ideas and look for a more adequate solution to elevate the house above the paradigms of domestic architecture of the time, bringing a new thought to the cultural conditions of the moment (Sikora, 2018).

At Maggie's, the co-clients constantly guide the architects—who are part of a larger *project team*—in responding to the seemingly simple, yet difficult to inter-pret, requests of the Architectural Brief. And while they help them in this difficult reading, the co-clients challenge them to go beyond the brief, even using some cognitive modalities. In this regard, Neurosciences confirm that meeting certain types of charismatic people could lead to a situation in which one feels dimin-ished or, conversely, empowered. "Being pushed into a leadership role may have brought out the best in you" (Damasio, 1994, p. 182). In fact, when I asked if any architect could design a Maggie's centre, even with the constant guidance of the co-clients, the architects responded: "Maybe in asking to design a Maggie's centre, they would bring out the best of the architects" (*Aabø, 02.11.2018*).

While everyone agrees that Maggie's is "the best client an architect could wish for", and although there is freedom in the Architectural Brief and it does not impose schemes or assumptions, the co-clients—now 'client-experts'—prove to have full control over every single detail of the building, so the architect occasionally com-plains, saying: "We enjoyed working with them, not because it was open and free and you could do anything, that's really not true" (*de Rijke, 17.12.2018*). On the other hand, the work of the co-clients, which has become exponentially complicated in recent years due to the growing number of centres and the difficulty of finding funds, is that of not losing sight of the final objective which is to satisfy the users' needs. Let's not forget that Laura Lee is a former nurse and she knows the needs of people with cancer very well. In fact, feeding heavily on visitors' opinion, when a new project starts, the *design team* confronts the cancer population, announcing the arrival of a new centre in town and showing what it will be like. Strategically, Mag-gie's co-clients involve the users of the new site and eventually form the 'Triad'.

And we listen. We already have extensive knowledge of what they might need, but to offer them this hope and to have a conversation early in the planning process, we invite local stakeholders to come in and see what we are doing and what we are planning.

(*Maggie's@Salus, 2021*)

With the opening of a new centre, for the co-clients, the new architect and new users, the research-design-construction process restarts. In an unusual position as a repeat client, compared to those clients who hire an architect only once and therefore cannot learn from him/her, Maggie's continually learns by commissioning similar buildings to different architects, thus gaining more and more experience, explaining why the co-clients are, indeed, 'client-experts'. As multi-centre builder Mike Coleman, of Sir Robert McAlpine Special Projects, said:

> Maggie's set up an ethos that flows down through construction projects. And I think anyone who is aware of construction projects, anything that is a cutting-edge design, anything that is trying to challenge the 'art of the possible', will have conflict, can have risk. And yet, Maggie's has this most amazing solution, which hasn't just delivered one Maggie's centre, but actually is a repeated delivery programme.
>
> (*Sir Robert McAlpine Special Projects@Salus, 2021*)

In this continuous learning process, the co-clients as well as the architects learn. When I asked the architects how useful this project was for them, David Page said: "Maggie's project has had a huge impact on our practice" (*Page, 01.10.2018*) and when I asked what they share and if Maggie's architects can be considered a community, Chris McVoy (SHA) said they share the experience of having done something important for humanity (*McVoy, 26.5. 2018*), while Piers Gough (*16.05.2018*) said that they are a community in the sense that "it is a bit like an architecture school" where everyone has left their mark and learned.

> And they left clear ideas and thoughts and maybe they will come back as a tutor. And you stand on their backs and then the next batches stand on your back and everyone learns from the previous one. So, in this way, we are a community.
>
> (*Gough, 16.05.2018*)

After learning and discussing architecture within the "Architecture, Art, Landscape and Flowers" category of the *Emotional* support programme, to which they have brought their experience and knowledge and from which they have acquired a strong sense of agency, Maggie's users also have a say, working to become 'user-experts'.

Within the theory of the 'Commissioning of Architecture' Maggie's provides a new contribution thanks to the uniqueness of Maggie's Triad—governed by an equally unique Architectural Brief—which, thanks to an active learning and the wealth of knowledge of the three components, is able to develop a real "Art of Commissioning". To understand the degree of success and become a model, as we will again see in Chapter 7, it is necessary to consider all the figures of Maggie's Triad, for the benefit of other projects and other triads.

The Co-Clients

From 1996 onwards, Charles Jencks, Laura Lee and Marcia Blakenham played the role of Maggie's *Architecture Co-Clients*, tasked not with "dictating the architecture" but rather "influencing the feeling, which then influences the architecture" (*Lee, 18.05.2019*). After Charles' death on 7 October 2019, Laura and Marcia continued their mission alone. Coming, as mentioned, from a nursing background in the NHS—where windows in hospital spaces are assumed to be unimportant (Marsh, 2018)—and without an architectural knowledge, Laura Lee had to educate herself, surprising many people, including her staff and other clients, who didn't really believe that architecture could help.

According to Laura Lee, the client's job is to keep architects focused on the architecture and its ultimate goal, which is "how to make people feel". This unusual way of instructing architects derives from the emotional Architectural Brief. "The whole point is that if you give someone a technical brief, that means that people say: 'I will just deliver that technical requirement'" (*Lee, 18.05.2019*). By asking the architect to think deeply about what the purpose of the project is, vice versa, the co-clients will obtain a building that arouses emotions.

> I think that when we look at plans or drawings, the basic question underneath anything we ask is: what is going to feel like for someone who is going to use it? So, we try not to talk about aesthetics, but it's what is going to feel like to be used by somebody who is in a horrible moment, psychologically.
>
> (*Blakenham, 18.05.2019*)

Even more unusual is the way the two women guide the architect by not telling him/her what they want, but rather what they don't want. For example, they don't want people to feel manipulated or that the building hides secrets.

> So, we work from another point of view, of things that we don't want that people may feel: we don't want to make people feel processed; we don't want to make people feel like they are in a factory. So, we have that conversation rather than telling the architect what it is, because what you are telling is already restricting his/her creativity and freedom to find the solution for what it is.
>
> (*Lee, 18.05.2019*)

Maggie's contradictory nature begins to emerge from this quote. By telling the architect what they don't want, the 'client-experts' get what they want, demonstrating that the 'little said' helps to identify the role of those few written words or rules contained in the Architectural Brief. However, since it is not the client's goal to theorise and make "assumptions on how the person entering the door must feel", in the end, the co-clients deliberately leave the architect free. Indeed, it is in the free interpretation of the white space 'between the lines' that the true recipe for Maggie's success lies.

Another thing about Maggie's co-clients that might seem unusual to a regular client is not expecting perfection from the architect.

> And I think, weirdly, all our buildings may have imperfections, many imperfections, but they don't matter. We don't mind too much, as long as the feelings are right. We keep going back to this thing about feelings. If the feeling is right, you can take the overall.
>
> (*Blakenham, 18.05.2019*)

Among the 'imperfections' mentioned by Laura Lee is that of acoustics, a problem that we find in all Maggie's centres as a consequence of the open space required by the Architectural Brief. As Laura Lee says, in a mentality of adaptability and flexibility, the problem of acoustics must be taken as an asset rather than an imperfection, as, indeed, all imperfections should be taken. And, even if for some people this is not the case, since visitors are all different and not everyone sees or hears the same, it is up to them whether to accept it as a compromise—as they often do—and the proof of this is that even the most private conversations take place in the open and visible space. The transmission of sound, in fact, helps visitors feel they are a part of the community.

> If you still hear voices behind the walls, it means that you are not alone in the building, but that there is a community out there, of which you are a fundamental part.
>
> (*Lee, 09.03.2018*)

One last unusual thing about Maggie's co-clients is that they don't ask for urgent deadlines. Since Maggie's is a private organisation, the co-clients have time and are never in a hurry, because they know that if they rush the architect, he or she can make mistakes.

> And these mistakes are always the client's mistakes, never the architects. Beauty comes first. Only if you have a concept-free mind can you get the magic Maggie wanted.
>
> (*Lee, 09.03.2018*)

What the co-clients share with the architect is their ultimate goal, which is to acquire the ability to inspire people with cancer to react and to bring out something they had inside that they didn't know they had, feeling they can let go and be themselves.

> In the most vulnerable moment of their life, we want visitors to be able to enter a space and feel stimulated, explore what they may not dare to seek in another environment.
>
> (*Lee, 18.05.2019*)

Inviting the architects to investigate what Maggie's 'social challenge' is with cancer—which is a "very difficult job to do"—the co-clients ask the architect to go beyond the expected response to the client's call.

> And they have to do that hard lift, themselves. And we try to work with them and lift them hard and then we work to keep them exploring if they got it.
>
> (*Lee, 18.05.2019*)

Part of the learning process that the co-clients expect from the architect who has just been commissioned to build a new Maggie's centre is to visit existing centres. Indeed, this is another challenge raised by the co-clients, as there are now so many buildings that there is a risk that the new architect will be influenced. For example, Ivan Harbour (RSHP) developed his design idea before visiting Maggie's Edinburgh—according to him, "the real matrix of it all"—because he didn't want to be influenced. Conversely, some architects went to see many buildings without reading much of the Architectural Brief, because they felt they would learn more by seeing it applied in reality. For the co-clients, visiting existing centres also creates an opportunity to talk to the users and spend time with them in the space, as well as being an incentive to try and do better.

> I prefer to encourage when architects want to go and look at other buildings, because the right ones want to know what people think works and what doesn't.
>
> (*Blakenham, 18.05.2019*)

The Architects

Although history, as we have seen, demonstrates that the architect cannot achieve much without an inspired client (De Carlo, 2004) and since, often, an architect is considered more interested in the design of his building than in who will use it, the role of an attentive and thoughtful architect is essential to respond to the client's needs.

> An architect, by definition, is someone who cares. There is no question about that. There is no financial remuneration that will ever pay a care of an architect, it's just not. So, in a way, Maggie's philosophy was 'let's get all these architects who care to do it'.
>
> (*Page, 01.10.2018*)

Within the client–architect relationship, from the interviews I conducted with 12 of Maggie's architects to understand how they interpreted the Architectural Brief and clarify their design approach, a very high level of collaboration and encouragement emerged.

> They want you to think grandly. They remind me of the De' Medici family. They are the sponsors of *excellence* and *beauty*, what more can you ask for? So, they make you perform beyond yourself.
>
> (*Page, 01.10.2018*)

Confirming what has already been said, this relationship centres on freedom.

> What is amazing about this client is that they give architects freedom. Not many clients do that; the tendency is to correct the architects. In this case, the architects had the freedom.
>
> (*van Loon, 15.05.2018*)

> What is fascinating is that 'what do you think we ought to do?' and they are very open to that. If anything pushes you to be more like yourself and less like them. They are always very open to ideas.
>
> (*Gough, 16.05.2018*)

In the dialogue that the architect has with the co-clients, trust and respect are the basis, especially in budget management. In this, the architect is the first to want the interest of the client, but above all that of the users, knowing that the money comes from donations often collected by local communities.

> They are very experienced clients, and they are critical, but in a way that is constructive. So, we worked really closely with them and they were very critical in a good way. They were quite good at identifying what might be worth spending on and what might not. There isn't enough money and there isn't an opportunity to be indulgent inappropriate in any way with such a project. Yet, there is trust and that's a very special thing to work with, between a client and an architect. So, trust and respect were two ways and that doesn't always happen with projects. Sometimes architects are regarded with a certain amount of suspicion, because typically they can spend a lot of money when it is not necessary.
>
> (*de Rijke, 17.12.2018*)

The architect will soon discover that the most important challenge launched by the co-clients is to 'dare', which is completely unusual in the world of professional practice. Typically, architects are obsessed with the idea that the client can ask them to make changes, perhaps distorting the project, while maintaining the same budget.

> And Charlie and Laura came to my office, and they said 'No, no. We want your signature, the 'green tile', that's what we want! We want what you did at that lavatories in Westbourne Grove, we want that look, we want that feel of ceramic'. So 'fine, ok!' And I was like 'Can we afford it?' 'For Goodness' sake… Don't worry about it! We don't want to build a building less good, because we are trying to economise, that's not the way we work. It's not our thinking!'
>
> (*Gough, 16.05.2018*)

In response to the co-clients' briefing, the architect begins working on the project, developing the usual themes of a therapeutic space (nature, comfort, sense of refuge, etc.), with customised solutions that will eventually lead to a 'superb' product. For Maggie's architects, nature is not a 'theme', but a real 'material'. For Ellen van Loon (OMA), at Maggie's Glasgow (2011) the garden was, in fact, the most important material: "The great idea was to bring nature into the building made of concrete and glass" (*16.05.2018*). For Alex de Rijke and Jasmin Sohi (dRMM) at Maggie's Oldham (2017) it was not just about bringing nature inside the building with a silver birch in the centre, but the whole building wanted to express the connection between nature and health. Built over a garden open to the entire hospital, the first permanent construction in the UK using the CLT (Cross Laminated Timber) technique—also economical because it is supplied in a 'kit' which allows for rapid construction—it is carbon dioxide free, resulting in a building that is healthy in itself and therapeutic for its users.

These sorts of solutions made me think that Maggie's architects had a particular specialist experience of healing architecture. Yet, no. As explained in Chapter 2, none of the 12 architects I spoke to had any technical experience of healing architecture. Indeed, David Page, author of Maggie's Glasgow the Gatehouse (2002) and Maggie's Highlands (2005), said: "I struggle with the notion of scientific proof. I think that if we had waited for scientific knowledge nothing would have ever happened" (*Page, 01.10.2018*). Ivan Harbour, author of Maggie's West London (2008), also added:

> As architects the idea of being a specialist is an anathema really, because specialists know the answer, but as an architect you don't want to know the answer, you need to find the answer with your client, or an answer.
>
> (*Harbour, 20.07.2018*)

Among the previous studies on the Maggie's centre, the theme of scientific knowledge of healing architecture had already been addressed by Van der Linden, Annemans and Heylighen (2015, 2016), who had also highlighted the need to transfer knowledge directly from users to designers because "a lack of direct user engagement introduces the risk of an unrealistic user image" (2016, p. 531). Reflecting at length on their conclusions, namely that the design of the Maggie's centre is not based on scientific knowledge but on an intuitive and personal participation of the architect—which will eventually lead him/her to create a building that evokes the emotional states required by the Brief—I realised that, as we will see in Chapter 7, being a very profound human experience, the project of a Maggie's centre emotionally involves architects to such an extent that they not only go beyond the brief, but they go beyond themselves. This means that not only visitors feel facilitated in acting guided by their own emotional state, but also the emotionally involved architect undergoes a cognitive process that helps him/her generate his/her project, ultimately confirming Damasio's theory according to which feelings and emotions govern reasoning and decision-making.

> It is as if we are possessed by a passion for reason, a drive that originates in the brain core, permeates other levels of the nervous system, and emerges as either feelings or nonconscious biases to guide decision making.
>
> (Damasio, 1994, p. 245)

The Users: Staff and Visitors

Maggie's users are the third tip of the Triad and being those who experience the building every day (staff) or during their visits (visitors), they are a fundamental component of it. Generally speaking, within the provision of services to the public such as those of hospitality, welfare or healthcare, we know that there are always two types of users, complementary but adverse, who usually use the building in an antithetical way: 'staff' and 'guests', 'employees' and 'assisted', 'nurses' and 'patients'. In particular, in the healthcare sector, nurses and patients receive very different perceptions from the environment and have totally opposite experiences, most often both of dissatisfaction. These different perceptions derive both from the underlying philosophy of the organisation or institution and from the architectural conformation of the environment.

At Maggie's these two aspects coincide. As already seen, the open and continuous spaces required by the Brief—which, on the other hand, bans 'spaces reserved for staff only'—facilitate the work of the staff who, through the support programme, promote participation and a 'being with them'. In fact, when entering a Maggie's centre it is difficult to distinguish between the staff and the visitors because, despite the different health conditions, the two categories of users occupy the same spaces and behave in the same way to the point that we can consider them as a single category. The fact that the staff do not wear a uniform or do not use a specific language certainly helps as does the fact that both types of users play an active role.

With more time on their hands than they had in the hospital—where they were perpetually under pressure—Maggie's staff are always available to visitors and do so with apparent ease, even if, at times, it can be psychologically exhausting. Since, the staff is very skilled at not showing it and at making everyone feel calm and relaxed, visitors think that the staff are very happy, also because "they work in a beautiful environment". Furthermore, visitors believe that guiding the staff 'from above', with precise rules, is Maggie's strategy to make visitors feel equally guided and, therefore, reassured that they are in good hands.

> Like a child who expects his or her parent to behave calmly, visitors expect the same from the staff and this is what allows us to have a strong sense of control.
>
> (*Focus-group Barts*)

Becoming a good staff member, however, is not an easy or straightforward path. With a background in a very disciplined work in the healthcare sector, usually carried out in confined spaces, lacking natural light and quality, new staff members—unlike visitors who rarely dislike the building at first glance—often don't understand Maggie's open and undefined spaces and struggle to 'surrender' to the building. Considering that, among the staff, volunteers rotate quite often, but that they are also the ones with the primary role of offering the 'cup of tea', it is important that this adaptation process happens quickly. Fortunately, time helps to familiarise and soon the staff begins to appreciate the space: in a domino effect, as Charles Jencks used to say, the building supports the staff who, in turn, supports the visitors (2015, p. 10).

Thanks to the synergistic work done by the building and the staff in promoting the motto 'empower the patient' and the 'help-yourself' strategy, as mentioned, Maggie's visitors are called to contribute, a way for people with cancer to react to the passive state inflicted on them when they were patients in the hospital and to take an active role in the community that makes them feel like normal people.

> You put the glass away and put it in the dishwasher. So, you take something and then clean up after yourself, which is important. (…) So, here it's the freedom that just says you can do yourself.
>
> (*Follow-up Barts*)

In addition to the practical contribution, visitors, already 'user-experts' of architecture, feel they can contribute by suggesting ideas to the *design team* to improve the quality of the experience of the space.

> It's not an insult to say this [the problem with acoustics] to the architect, it's just that; when he or she does the next building or when the next Maggie's is built, they have to take that into account. That's all.
>
> (*Focus-group Barts*)

Free to have their say, sometimes Maggie's visitors (men more than women) know how to be very critical and express their opinion in no uncertain terms. At Maggie's Dundee, during the focus group with the men's group, it emerged that Grayson Parry's painting, the *Print for Politician* (1999), hanging at the back of the large sitting room, aroused mixed feelings and many found it disturbing. This brings us back to the sense of provocation Charles Jencks described when he spoke about Zaha Hadid's architecture. According to Jencks, this is how we should think of 'hospital art' "as a provocation and not as a consolation" (Jencks and Heathcote, 2010, p. 29). But male visitors at Maggie's Dundee disagree on the 'provocation' aspect and have called for the painting to be removed.

> You could put it in a museum, and I would look at it, but being in this room for the purpose we are in this room is not relevant. We use adjectives like 'familiar' and 'comforting' and in a supportive and welcoming environment you would

expect to apply none of them to a picture like this. It's challenging, but there are enough challenging things that happen in your life if you're here; you don't need them, you don't even want to see them. Actually, this image is depressing. So, maybe there is something worse in life. Well, this picture is worse than what we have, but is this what we need? No, I don't think so.

(Focus-group_no.1 Dundee)

At Maggie's, users from different backgrounds, with all sorts of stories, can be very eloquent about their ideas, but more importantly they have the freedom to express them and can tell architects what works and what doesn't. As we shall see in Chapter 7, by strengthening their position within Maggie's Triad, visitors share the feelings the building arouses in them and make their contribution to the *design team*. As Maggie's teaches, it is therefore essential to give users a voice.

References

Alexander, C., Ishikawa, S. and Silverstein, M. (1977) *A Pattern Language: Towns, Buildings, Construction.* New York: Oxford University Press

Barrett, P. and Stanley, C. (1999) *Better Construction Briefing.* Oxford: Blackwell Science

BBC (2016) 'Building Hope: The Maggie's Centres', Full BBC Documentary. https://www.youtube.com/watch?v=QkVcZuAikrI&t=2083s&ab_channel=nomadwariror

Blakenham, M. (2007) 'Foreword and Maggie's Centres: Marching on', in Keswick M. (1994) *A View from the Front Line.* https://maggies-staging.s3.amazonaws.com/media/filer_public/5b/f6/5bf6f8c7-37e4-4b0a-b09d-6ad48d66387d/view-from-the-front-line.pdf

Blyth, A. and Worthington, J. (2007) *Il progetto e il committente. La pratica del briefing per la gestione del processo progettuale.* Italian edition by Carlotta Fontana (ed). Naples: Esselibri

Brennan, S. (2015) 'Patterns of Neurons Firing'. Interview with Sabina Brennan. Interviewed by N. McLaughlin and Y. Manolopoulou for Losing Myself http://www.losing-myself.ie/pages/patterns-neurons-firing/

Damasio, A. (1994) *Descartes' Error: Emotion, Reason, and the Human Brain.* London: Vintage

Damasio, A. (2000) *The Feeling of What Happens. Body, Emotion and the Making of Consciousness.* London: Vintage

Damasio, A. (2004) *Looking for Spinoza. Joy, Sorrow and the Feeling Brain.* London: Vintage

Folador, M. (2006) *L'organizzazione perfetta. La regola di San Benedetto. Una saggezza antica al servizio dell'impresa moderna.* Milan: Guerini e Associati

Fontana, C. (2007) 'Utilità del brief: analisi delle esigenze e organizzazione del processo', in Blyth, A. and Worthington, J. (eds.) "Il progetto e il committente. La pratica del briefing per la gestione del processo progettuale". Italian edition by Carlotta Fontana (ed). Naples: Esselibri, pp. 13–19

Howells, L. (2016) 'Synergy between People and Place', TEDxTalks. https://www.youtube.com/watch?v=tvE78D30CbQ

Jencks, C. (2015) *The Architecture of Hope: Maggie's Cancer Caring Centres* (2nd ed.). London: Frances Lincoln

Jencks, C. and Heathcote, E (2010) *The Architecture of Hope: Maggie's Cancer Caring Centres.* London: Frances Lincoln

Kearney, M. (2009) *A Place of Healing: Working with Nature & Soul at the End of Life.* New Orleans: Spring Journal Books

Keswick, M. (1994) 'A View From The Frontline'. Revised and reprinted in 2003 and 2007. https://maggies-staging.s3.amazonaws.com/media/filer_public/5b/f6/5bf6f8c7-37e4-4b0a-b09d-6ad48d66387d/view-from-the-front-line.pdf

Maggie's Brief (2015) 'Architectural and Landcape Brief'. https://maggies-staging.s3.amazonaws.com/media/filer_public/e0/3e/e03e8b60-ecc7-4ec7-95a1-18d9f9c4e7c9/maggies_architecturalbrief_2015.pdf

Marsh, H. (2018) 'Why are Hospitals so often Horrible?' Speaker for the Phil Gusack Talk at the AfH AGM at RIBA, 22 February. https://www.slideshare.net/Architectsforhealth/henry-marsh-phil-gusack-talk-at-riba-feb-2018

Masterman, J. W. E. (1992) *Building Procurement System.* London: Spon

Salisbury, F. (1998) *Briefing Your Architect.* London and New York: Routledge

Salvatorelli, L. (1983) *San Benedetto e l'Italia del suo tempo.* Rome-Bari: Ed. Laterza

Santacroce, R. (2015) *L'architetto e il Committente. Il processo di briefing come strumento per l'architettura.* Copyrights MUD Architects. https://issuu.com/m.u.d.architects/docs/l_architetto_e_il_committente

Sikora, S. (2018) 'Willey House Stories Part 5. The Best of Clients', Frank Lloyd Wright Foundation. https://franlloydwright.org/willey-house-stories-part-5-the-best-of-clients/

Suárez De La Torre, E. (2005) 'Il mito e il culto di Asclepio in Grecia in età classica ed el-lenistico romana', in De Miro, E., Sfameni Gasparro, G. and Calì, V. (eds.) "Il culto di Asclepio nell'area mediterranea". Rome: Giangemi Editore.

Van der Linden, V., Annemans, M. and Heylighen, A. (2016) 'Architects' Approaches to Healing Environment in Designing a Maggie's Cancer Caring Centre', *The Design Journal*, 19(3), pp. 511–533

Yu, A. T. W., Qiping, Shen, Q., Kelly, J. and Hunterb, K. (2007) 'An Empirical Study of the Variables Affecting Construction Project Briefing/Architectural Programming', *International Journal of Project Management*, 25(2), pp. 198–212

Zwemmer, M. and den Otter, A. (2008) 'Engaging Users in Briefing and Design: A Strategic Framework', *Semantic Scholar*, pp. 405–421

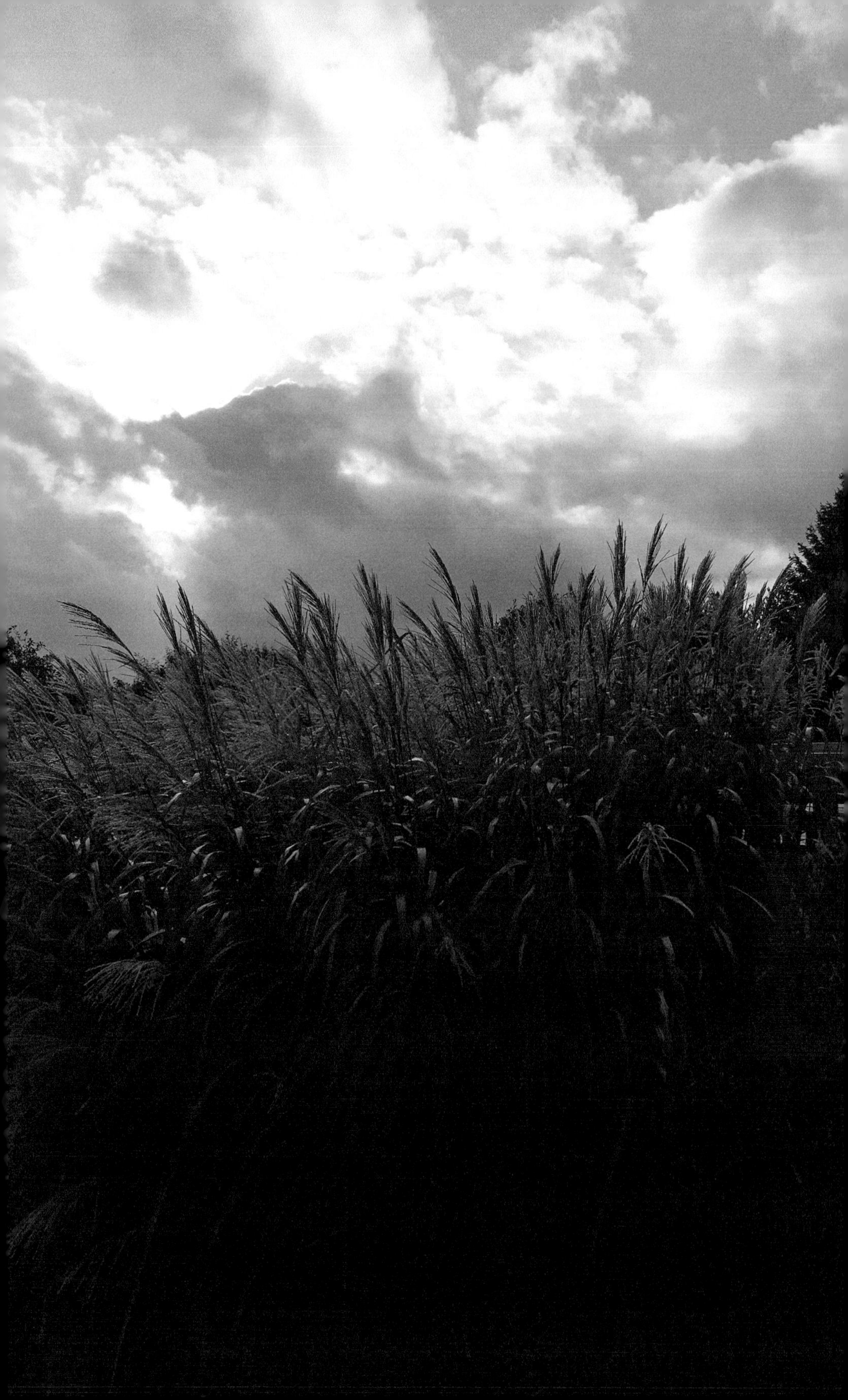

5

MAGGIE'S SYNERGY

Synergy between People and Place

The term 'synergy' derives from the Greek word συνεργός (*synergos*) which means 'to work together' (Cambridge Dictionary, 2023). Although Aristotle never used it, in his *Metaphysics* he wrote:

> In the case of all things which have several parts and in which the totality is not, as it were, a mere heap, but the whole is something besides the parts, there is a cause; for even in bodies contact is the cause of unity in some cases, and in others viscosity or some other such quality.
>
> (Aristotle, 350 BC)

Throughout history, the concept of 'synergy' has been used in various disciplines. In Theology, Edward Reynolds (1599–1676), bishop of Norwich, mentioned the words "synergy and co-partnership with Christ and with God" to describe the co-operation of human effort with the Divine Will (Chalmers, 1826, p. 158). Later in history, the taken-for-granted authorless axiom "synergy is the creation of a whole that is greater than the simple sum of its parts" was used in physics, biochemistry, science and psychology. In the 1920s, 'synergy' became the motto of Gestalt Psychology according to which the perception of reality allowed the individual to grasp something more than the totality of the parts of the object (Koffka, 1935). As we shall see in the next chapter, in the context of Merleau-Ponty's Phenomenology, this same 'totality' is called 'structure'—in fact, the lifeworld has a meaningful structure of its own (Wild, 1962, xiii)—"whose properties are not the sum of those which the isolated parts would possess" (Merleau-Ponty, 1963 [1942], p. 47). At Maggie's, this 'totality' is generated by the open and hybrid space made

DOI: 10.4324/9781003244516-5

up of the "many things" that Maggie desired and to which people with cancer are called to access.

In a social behavioural context, the notion of 'synergy' is defined as the combined power of a group of individuals that is greater and more efficient when work is done collaboratively rather than individually (Bratton et al., 2008). This is true even if the combination occurs between humans and artefacts, something that Jacobs (2006) calls "building events", assemblages of human and non-humans. In this regard, as mentioned in Chapter 2, in his studies on the Maggie's centre, Daryl Martin (2016) had already advanced the hypothesis of a synergism between people and place, improved by the presence of objects and furniture scattered around the centre, essential for creating a familiar environment (Martin, 2016, 2017), enhanced by "generators of architectural atmospheres" i.e. the combination of materials, light, colour and shape of buildings (Martin, Nettleton and Buse, 2019).

> Working in tandem with the architecture, professional staff and volunteers are key to establishing the atmospherics of care in a Maggie's centre, and their work includes elements of curating and cultivating the spaces within which that care is experienced.
>
> (Martin, 2016, p. 40)

Lesley Howells (2016) built her hypothesis on this intuition: the coexistence of people in a stimulating place like Maggie's bright kitchen, where the large table invites "therapeutic conversations" (Martin, 2014), helps people to open up and accept the support offered, even when the staff is absent.

> It's a natural fact: if you can place somebody in the building, they can actually achieve very similar results to mine with talk therapy.
>
> (*Howells, 16.06.2017*)

Within the concept of 'synergy between people and place', according to Architectural Phenomenology the *place* is a necessary but insufficient condition without the human presence that not only interacts with the place, but 'dwells' or 'inhabits' it (Heidegger, 1971 [1954]; Relph, 1976; Seamon and Mugerauer, 1985), giving rise to the concept of the "man-in-the-world" or "individual-in-his-habitat". This idea originated in the biological concept of *Umwelt* (=surrounding world) developed by Jakob von Uexküll (1926), according to whom all organisms effectively construct their environment by selecting the characteristics with which they can interact. Since *habitat*, from the Latin verb *habeo* (=to have), in the frequentative form 'continue to have' is something that we carry with us and to which we refer when everything around us collapses (D'Avenia, 2018) and, as *individuals,* from the Latin term *individuus* (=undivided) we are inseparable from our own characteristics (i.e. our individuality), which make us unique and therefore different from any other, if we want to in-habit-the-place, the *place* must offer 'many solutions' so that each individual can, within the 'whole', find the right spot that adapts to his/her mood of the moment. In a Maggie's centre, within the 'spatial interaction rather than walls', the offer of multiple solutions is what activates the 'synergy between people and place', generating the feeling, as Harbour (RSHP) argues, that the space is divided, but at the same time connected.

> I think the openness, the interconnection between the slightly loosely defined spaces is a way of generating a little buzz in the atmosphere that makes you think that you are part of a bigger enterprise, but without it being, or feeling like you're in one big room. That's the subtle distinction and I think that is probably one of the core things that Maggie's talked about, this idea that you don't feel, you should never feel, as if you can't go anywhere within the building. In other words, it should not be a series of rooms, although at the same time it needs to have rooms, the ability to have rooms, but without feeling as if there are rooms that are not for you.
>
> (*Harbour, 20.07.2018*)

As for the *people*, according to Human Geography, through the "bodily connection with architecture", the bodies are moved by the buildings that orchestrate the movements inside them "supplying the perceptive body with a set of possible actions or movements to perform" (Kraftl and Adey 2008, p. 227). Furthermore, the materiality of architecture generates the sensory "feel" of a building and is concerned with "affective, tactile, sensual effects" (2008, p. 214). From this theory, we can deduce—and confirm—that the link with the architecture is established through movement, and that our senses are stimulated by materials "held together" in specific assemblages. These two aspects are central to how we choose the buildings we like to stay in. Indeed, there is an *a priori* 'selectivity' that depends on our affective relationship with another subject, in this case an architecture. The Maggie's centre generates such an affective relationship among its users that the same adjectives used for people (loving, cuddly, supportive) are used for the building. Only by considering the building ('the non-human') as an "occupied performative event" (Jacobs, 2006, p. 10), can we understand why Maggie's visitors, in addition to considering the building as a 'member of staff', feel for it an affection that you would feel for a friend.

> I suppose, in my mind, I think 'wow, I am valuable. I have got a creepy disease, I have it, I have been cured, I hope, whatever cancer, but I am valued'. So, this building says: 'you are valued, we care about you', you know, really very basic things. 'Hey, we love you, we want you'.
>
> (*Focus-group Barts*)

To understand this symbiotic affective relationship, we must consider that all events and places influence our cognitive and sensory experiences which are all, to some extent, imbued with affectivity; in other words, there is no such thing as 'non-affective thought' (Duncan and Feldman Barrett, 2007). At Maggie's, once immersed in the space, without realising it, visitors develop a cognitive process on a personal level stimulated by affective thoughts that allow the individual openness and flexibility.

Psychological Flexibility: The Fundamental Role of Architecture

We almost never think of the present, and when we do, it is only to see what light it throws on our plans for the future.

(Pascal, 1670, quoted by Damasio, 1994, p. 165)

So wrote Pascal, taken up by Damasio (1994) to tell us how little we share in our present moment, of which he even says that when we talk about it, it has already passed, indeed "the present is never here" (Damasio, 1994, p. 240). On the contrary, trying to detach from the past and focus on the "here and now" (Harris, 2013, p. 32), together with balancing future fears and desires, Steve Hayes and Smith (2005), help us understand how psychological flexibility and resilience, in times of uncertainty, constitute the ability to regulate emotions, a constant transaction between the individual and the context in which he/she moves (Kashdan & Rottenburg, 2010). By stopping and knowing how to bear difficult thoughts and emotions lightly, we are able to respond to unexpected changes in life and to fully live in the moment.

> Psychological flexibility means contacting the present moment fully as a conscious human being, and based on what the situation affords, changing or persisting in behaviour in the service of chosen values.
>
> (Hayes, 2021, para. 2)

Psychological Flexibility concerns the ability to act in accordance with what is most important to us, along with what the present situation offers us. It refers to the process by which individuals respond to changes arising from problematic situations and employ their mental resources to adjust their perspectives to new conditions. It is also a fundamental skill—as we learn from the second part of Hayes' definition "changing or persisting in behaviour in the service of chosen values"— that of knowing how to accept difficult thoughts or emotions in order to turn towards our values. And every time we turn to our values or anything that matters, we know we're going to have difficult thoughts and emotions.

Psychological Flexibility is not a talent or a trait one is born with, but rather a way of responding to events, a way of maintaining guidance in our existence based on skills that can be learned and practiced. Nor is it a way to avoid suffering as it is inevitably part of the human experience. As already seen in Chapter 4, since the dawn of existence, suffering has served to protect our survival, by increasing our attention to pain signals coming from the body proper and correcting the consequences, as well as "early body signals, in both evolution and development, contributed to forming a 'basic concept' of self" (Damasio, 1994, p. 240). In a stimulating environment, when people understand that they have a 'context of self', or the ability to stay in touch with a 'perspective of self' that does not vary according to transient emotions or thoughts, a sense of flexibility arises (Hayes, 2017).

Rooted in ACT (Acceptance and Commitment Therapy), which is part of the "third wave in behavioural and cognitive therapies" (Hayes and Smith, 2005, p. 2), Psychological Flexibility is both acceptance and commitment. Acceptance is fundamental because the opposite, i.e. attempting to free oneself from difficult thoughts and emotions, actually increases their frequency, intensity and duration (Hayes and Smith, 2005, p. 3).

> (...) 'accepting' the suffering linked to thoughts, emotions and unpleasant memories does not mean resigning oneself or giving them pleasure, but it means to stop investing energy in behaviours that do not work in the long run, and turn us away from life as we wanted it (...) Accepting serves only to free your hands from a useless struggle, to be able to engage them in other places, in other areas where you can build something significant and important.
>
> (Harris, 2013, pp. 37–38)

Commitment is equally important. Unlike other healthcare programmes where patients may not continue to participate, Maggie's psychologists work to engage visitors and make them feel committed. In a 2017 article, Charles Jencks reported on a phone call made in May–July 2016 with Lesley Howells—then Centre Head of Maggie's Dundee—during which Lesley was trying to convince Charles that what Maggie's does is adopt the 'self-help' mode to keep visitors busy so that they will come back next time and take part in further activities. "It is their commitment to variable and continuing self-help that is sustaining" (Jencks, 2017, p. 75).

The different stages of ACT/Psychological Flexibility are illustrated by a hexagonal model called *hexaflex*, which implies that the six steps ('acceptance', 'defusion', 'contact with the present moment', 'self-as-context', 'values' and 'committed actions') are strongly connected to each other and in fact inseparable, just like the six faces of a diamond (Harris, 2009, p. 30). The *hexaflex* model, however, can be represented in the simpler three-stage triangular *triplex* model of the three stages 'open-up', 'be present', 'do what matters' (Harris, 2009) (Figure 5.1A and 5.1B).

Keeping in mind the principle of *inclusion* underlying Maggie's synergy, by applying the three steps of the *triplex* model to the architecture of the three Maggie's centres of my ethnographic work, I was able to confirm the veracity of Howells'

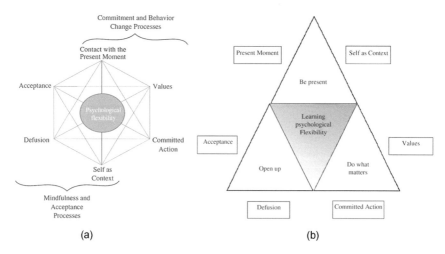

FIGURE 5.1A AND 5.1B The *hexaflex* and *triflex* models of Psychological Flexibility (Courtesy of Steven Hayes).

postulate "the synergy between people and place enables psychological flexibility" (*16.06.2017*) also from an architectural point of view.

1 "Opening up to reality" means accepting the choices that are offered to us.
  The open and continuous space of Maggie's kitchen helps people open up to social interactions and different types of conversations. In his design for Maggie's Dundee, Frank Gehry said he was inspired by the Yiddish concept of *heymish* (=familiarity, intimacy, safety) that the architecture expresses through the use of warm materials, large south-facing windows overlooking nature, intimate but open spaces that allow private but visible and therefore reassuring conversations. These physical conditions have an emotional impact on people which encourages them to take the lead. And since "everyone knows what to do in the kitchen" (Howells, 2016, 7:16), it is easy for new visitors to make a cup of tea, sit down and have a conversation with old visitors sharing experiences with them. This means that Maggie's synergy "allows someone to turn towards reality rather than struggle against it" (Howells, 2016, 0:45) (Figure 5.2).
2 "Being present with life as it is" means fully engaging in the current situation.
  Maggie's sensory space helps people to be fully present. At Maggie's Barts, Steven Holl was inspired by the colourful musical notations discovered in the nearby St. Bartholomew Church, which we find reinterpreted in the translucent glass facade dotted with coloured figures that recall Rothko's art. The positive atmosphere made of filtered light and colour that fills the large double-height open space—"because light transmits energy" (*McVoy, 05.26.2018*)—and collaborates with the large sculptural staircase, entices visitors in their climb, keeping them in action and in contact with reality. Enveloping them in an extraordinary multisensory experience, the architectural space detaches visitors

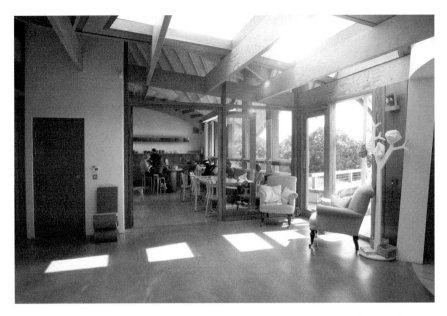

FIGURE 5.2 Maggie's kitchen helps people open-up to social interactions and 'therapeutic conversations' (Maggie's Dundee, 2003) (Courtesy of Maggie's).

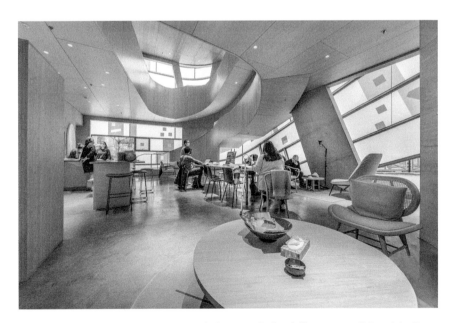

FIGURE 5.3 Maggie's sensory space helps people be fully present (Maggie's Barts, 2017) (©Marco Castelli Nirmal).

from their difficult thoughts and emotions and makes them appreciate the present moment. This means that Maggie's synergy allows someone to commit to the 'here and now' concept rather than being caught up in memories of the past or thoughts about the future (*Howells, 07.02.2019*) (Figure 5.3).

3 "Doing what matters to you" means acting according to our own values.

As Charles Jencks said, Maggie's icons help people to distract themselves, but also to focus on what is important to them and to act with commitment. In his design for Maggie's Oldham, Alex de Rijke drew inspiration from the stilted pavilion and, clearing the ground underneath and transforming it into a garden, he raised his building on poles and placed a silver birch in the centre. Enclosed in a full-height curved transparent glass case, the 'tree of life'—as the staff calls it to focus visitors' attention on 'what matters'— symbollically embodies the values that people recognise in it and offers them an inner perspective. This means that Maggie's synergy allows someone to find values not only externally but also internally, in the way they think about themselves, which can eventually be shared and become valuable to others (*Howells, 07.02.2019*) (Figure 5.4).

As in Asclepian Healing, in which the sick faced suffering tolerated thanks to the care of the *therapeutes* and the magnificent natural environment, in the three phases of psychological flexibility, Maggie's visitors go through difficult thoughts and emotions, bearable thanks to the care of the staff offering the support programme

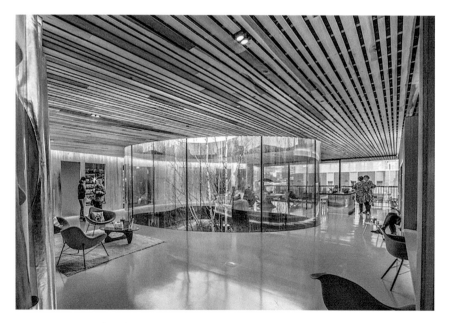

FIGURE 5.4 Maggie's icons distract but also help people focus on what's important to them and act with commitment (Maggie's Oldham, 2017) (©Marco Castelli Nirmal).

and the striking architecture that will accompany their minds in moving with "whatever is happening in their life". As Hayes concludes: "The science of psychological flexibility says that when you are open, when you are aware, then you can connect with the possibility of caring and being and doing" (2017, 1:14:05).

Maggie's Five-Step Healing Process: The Participants' Voice

The journey of a cancer patient begins in an NHS Oncology Department when he/she receives the *diagnosis* that puts him or her in a state of shock. Borrowing slogans from Maggie's brochures and website to title each of the sections of the five-step healing process that takes place in a Maggie's centre—that is, how Maggie's visitors move from a state of shock to a state of stability—, in the following sections I give users a voice. Since in the first two stages the visitors are not yet strong enough to speak, the narration will begin with the staff who witness the shocked condition of the visitors when they come in. After explaining how they help them to move toward psychological stabilisation, however, from the third stage onwards, I pass the word to the 'people with cancer', and not to their family or friends, because they are the best spokespersons for their experiences and they want to have a say.

In this regard, with reference to the main dilemmas that ethical literature in the health field has found itself facing when it comes to 'people with cancer', classifying them as 'vulnerable' or 'survivors' or even 'warriors', we imply our personal fear or distress about this condition (Wolinsky, 2019). Friends and family, but also organisations and even ethics committees, often take charge of the protection of patients by deciding for them, thinking it was for their best. However, when the university's ethics committee strongly advised me to rely on 'family members' rather than 'Maggie's psychologists' when needed, it turned out to be a mistake. As the participants in my ethnographic work themselves argued, after the initial difficult moment, people with cancer no longer want to involve family members in their experience at Maggie's, nor do they want to be represented by them, because the family treats them as incapable of making decisions. Telling someone that they are vulnerable, that they have no say in the matter and that they must have a family member next to them to give their consent is actually totally against the ethical principle. Ultimately, the recommendation from the university's ethics committee was not the right one to make.

A good way to highlight the participants' voice in an ethnographic work is through the sharing of ideas and participatory research. Unfortunately, as emerges from the literature on the ethics of 'cancer', research in this field focuses on the disease (Wright et al., 2006) and not on other topics such as 'the architecture of cancer facilities'. In my experience, involving people with cancer on the subject of 'architecture', in addition to making people feel 'normal'—and therefore good—given their knowledge and experience, has helped to put them in a position of respect to the point that some Maggie's participants no longer wanted to remain anonymous. Since compared to other categories such as that of 'architects', that of 'people with cancer' is of a broader nature, especially from a human point of view, the feedback received from this category has been far richer than that received from the 'architectural' one.

By sharing an interest and attitude towards a way of understanding life, the partici-pants who will speak below are able to recognise a therapeutic environment, aware that architecture not only creates the built environment, but goes deeper into our con-sciousness, forming our sense of identity, reflecting who we are and what we want.

> In brief, the endless reactivation of updated images about our identity (a combi-nation of memories of the past and the planned future) constitutes a sizable part of the state of the self as I understand it.
>
> (Damasio, 1994, p. 239)

'Just Come In' (Permission) (CCS's Voice)

The first encounter with the Maggie's centre is always quite emotional. The staff say that when they walk through the door, visitors are scared and, as mentioned, often in shock. As mentioned in Chapter 3, people with cancer usually come with their families, because unlike the hospital from which they are excluded for privacy reasons, Maggie's includes the family. As the staff say, when they arrive at the centre for the first time, simply by entering the building and finding a different en-vironment that is overwhelming, new visitors often start crying. The staff are there to help them and invite them to share their feelings and concerns, telling them that "it's okay to cry" and giving them permission 'to be emotional'.

> It's the expression we use when we talk to them. We invite them to share what's going on, in a place which is very much in contrast with the atmosphere of the hospital. Over there everybody is so busy, they don't have time, and people don't engage and sometimes there's this reluctance to engage with everyone, because they've got so many tasks that they have to complete.
>
> (*CCS_no.2 Barts*)

Without understanding what is happening to them, once they have calmed down, the new visitors, a little embarrassed, will say "I don't know what it is", "I can't explain it". The staff say that despite receiving an invitation to be emotional, visi-tors tend to be surprised at their own behaviour. According to them, this invitation mixed with a comforting environment and a relaxing atmosphere leads to an emo-tion that seems to be the release of the tension accumulated in the hospital: just walking through the door, almost a return to a domestic and safe environment "for some people could mean instant tears" (*CCS_no.2 Barts*).

> I think people are more willing to let their guard down when they walk in. They enter here, so that kind of barriers that they might have put up, they let them down. And I think the space helps that, I'm sure the space helps that, because their feelings are a bit more relaxed, more likely to disclose things.
>
> (*CCS_no.1 Barts*)

All these difficult thoughts and tormented emotions occur in the entrance space—which, as we know, the Architectural Brief calls 'pause' space because it is where visitors take a moment to stop and think—and in the welcome area where newcomers 'meet' the space. The staff say visitors always take a 'deep breath' when they meet it, perhaps as a sign of acceptance.

> What I've noticed is that people, because there is the space, which is nice, they always take a breath. It's a chance for them to take a breath. And people do actually get quite emotional sometimes. And they might cry a little bit and they'll say: 'I don't know why I'm doing it'. And I haven't really said or it's anything that we've said or done particularly, but it's just this chance, maybe that's acceptance.
> (*CCS_no.1 Barts*)

The staff warmly welcomes newcomers explaining that at Maggie's they don't have to pay anything or provide their data and that everyone is free to do what they want; so, if they don't want to talk to anyone they don't have to, but if they want to socialise they just have to ask. Despite being told to "act like they're at home", new visitors are still too shy or respectful to take the initiative. "It's okay to have a drink". "Yes, really?" "Yes, please help yourself". The Cancer Support Specialist (CCS) says that, in this way, people gradually gain the confidence they need to make themselves a drink, although, in this opening process, the staff still has to be by their side to make them feel comfortable.

'Here with You' (Stabilisation) (Psychologist's Voice)

After the CCS has helped new visitors lower their level of fear in the entrance or welcome area, the psychologists explain that when they come to them, they may still be frightened. During counselling sessions, psychologists notice that for the new visitors there is much more to go through than they can actually do at the moment, and they realise that the visitors will not be able to do it on their own. Newcomers are under tremendous pressure and know that, in the midst of fear, they have to make decisions about a new experience that they often don't understand. And to make these decisions they need to be able to think about what's happening to them, and they can't.

> And so, *I am with them* from that point of feeling scared, scared because they're about to face something that they're not going to be able to cope with, if not supported. And I am with them from that point through, helping them, enabling them, and that's my task, to stabilise slightly, to start to scope the task of it.
> (*Psychologist Barts*)

Using the cognitive abilities of people with cancer as much as possible and placing 'freedom of choice' in people's hands to start making decisions, psychologists say that the stabilisation process begins almost immediately and opens up to flexibility.

> And it's surprising how – and I see it again and again and again – people face a situation they don't know how to cope or survive with and they do. Often what seemed insurmountable becomes possible for them.
>
> *(Psychologist Barts)*

Once they're a little firmer on their feet, thanks to Maggie's psychological support and other types of support that visitors may find elsewhere, psychologists say that they can work towards flexibility. People with cancer and their family are now in a better position to start seeing what is happening to them and psychologists facilitate this very slow process helping them to see reality, allowing them to understand their difficult thoughts and emotions.

But when exactly does the building come into play? At first people often do not realise that these are special buildings, because they are focused on themselves and their problems. But when they are no longer frightened and can see the people and the space around them, after the contribution of the CCS in the welcome area, and that of the psychologist in the consultation room, it will be the building that intervenes by inviting the new visitors to stay and telling them to keep coming.

> If it were an awful building, and I was seeing people just as individual appointments, people would not stay, since they don't have the space and time around the appointment, which is very important, and I might talk to people about that. I may say, you know, 'take your time afterwards, just sit on a bench here and look at the space and think what we've discussed', because that's part of it, you know, that does further work. I remember I saw somebody who came out and just stopped.
>
> *(Psychologist Barts)*

If, at the end of the session, people with cancer move from the consultation room to the open kitchen area and stay to have a cup of tea or, vice-versa, if they wait for their appointment in the welcome area before entering the consultation room, during that extra time spent in the space, the building impacts visitors for a sufficient period of time that will help them prepare to have a better state of mind or extends the benefit of psychological therapy.

> I think the building provides time and space and allows them to be with what they're going to discuss with me before they come in, because I have noticed that once inside, if they have been sitting for a while in a comfortable space that is for them—and I think the people do really feel that—the difference is beyond the description, really. I mean, no doubt about it, an extraordinary difference between that and being in a corridor or in lined up seats. And I think it allows people to be with others, to be with themselves and their problems in a place where they feel safe. I mean, it provides such safety.
>
> *(Psychologist Barts)*

Although to date not many imaging experiments have been conducted in neuroscientific laboratories in search of a physiological response to the emotional experience of architectural environments (Mallgrave, 2013), from what the staff reported, it emerged that, at Maggie's, visitors react to the intense pleasure coming from the space, first emotionally and then consciously. As we will see in Chapter 6, this is explained by neuroscience with the fact that, within the homeostatic mechanisms of the body, in a preconscious way that cannot be described ("I don't know what it is"), the emotion comes first and then, in a conscious and describable way, comes the feeling (Damasio, 2004).

'Everyone's Home of Cancer Care' (Adaptation/Safety) (Visitors' Voice)

After the first meeting with the CCS and the psychologist, while people with cancer continue to go to the hospital for treatments, people with cancer still don't or may not have much control. During treatments, they have to listen very carefully to what is happening, in an attempt to grasp what they are being told and to regulate themselves around that information. And it is not until they leave the hospital and arrive at Maggie's, as already seen in Chapter 3, that they feel safe, can regain control and are able to think.

> When I come here, control is part of me, but it's not when I'm down there [in the hospital] (…) and it's not until you come away, and you're in a safe environment that you can go back to, that you feel in control.
>
> *(Follow-up Dundee)*

This concept of a safe space, a space that allows visitors to work on their priorities at their own pace, is left to the individual: from sitting in a corner without talking to anyone to being in a peer support group discussing a particular type of cancer or need. Feeling safe, people are able to focus on their choices or share their emotions.

> When I first came in, I did not know where to go or what to do. After sitting there for a while, I was looking around and felt really contained. I don't know, it was the environment with bright light coming through a huge glass downstairs that have made it feel at home. And then suddenly someone was talking to me and it was like waking up and it just felt it was ok to speak about it. And it just made me feel safe. I'd say it calmed me, in a way, it made me see.
>
> *(Focus-group Barts)*

For some visitors I've met, Maggie's is not only a 'life saver' but also a 'relationship saver'.

> I couldn't believe my cancer diagnosis. But then I thought 'I can come here every day! I can sit in a corner and cry some time, yeah!' I swear to God, if

I didn't have it, I don't think I would be ok as I am. And I don't bombard my poor husband, my family. You know, you will say 'Oh I went to Maggie's' 'oh, how was it?' 'it was great'. And I have been probably sobbing for two hours.

(*Focus-group Barts*)

The next step for new visitors is to meet old visitors and start a conversation. The easiest place to do that is by the kitchen counter over a simple "pass me the milk". By preparing the drinks themselves, no longer as a permission but with the 'freedom' to help themselves, a sense of self-confidence begins to arise.

One of the things I quite like is that you can come in and make your own drinks. Yes, I quite like can we all just come in, make a cup of tea. It's the first thing I do when I come in, and the fact that you do it yourself.

(*Follow-up Barts*)

Perceived as coming from both the building and the staff, the invitation to feel free also means letting your emotions out; visitors will feel safe doing so, because they know it is their choice.

And if I just want to come in here, come upstairs or sit here and look outside the window, I can do that. Or if I want to go and sit in a chair downstairs and just let it all come out, I can do that as well. So, that's freedom, you have control, but you have the freedom to do that.

(*Follow-up Dundee*)

Everyone appreciates the view of nature and the ability to sit inside and look out and into the distance. Having experienced and understood the beneficial power of this effect, one of my participants, Anne, told me that, although she had "probably, at the most two or three years left to live", she wanted to submit an alteration and replicate the same window of Maggie's Dundee in her home. This would allow her not only to gain the view but, knowing how hard it was for her husband, also to find a way to help him with a window.

We've got a lovely cottage with a lovely garden but it's quite dark, very Scottish. And I can be outside, but when I don't feel well, I need to sit inside and have a view like this. So, we are about to submit an alteration in the upstairs room so to make a window. And for my husband this window will be his goal for me. I've never thought a window with a view was a priority.

(*Follow-up Dundee*)

At this stage visitors realise that the view from above or outward provides a sense of control. Appreciating the psychological effects released by the building, they begin to understand the role of architecture in creating a therapeutic environment but also in being a focus for life.

'You Are not the Only One' (Normalisation/Normality) (Visitors' Voice)

When they go to the hospital, people become patients by taking on a patient's personality and behaving as a patient. When they walk into a Maggie's centre, they stop acting like patients and suddenly go back to being themselves. In this, both the staff and the building remind visitors of who they are. As a consequence, even though the family still sees them as vulnerable, therefore 'not normal', people with cancer soon begin to fight back.

> And at Maggie's I just don't have to pretend like I have to do with my family. It's one of those things that you say to your family, but they are like: 'So somebody else got the same thing, because we all have to endure things', which is a nightmare. I find it so easy that I don't have to pretend here or hide, at all.
>
> (*Focus-group Barts*)

Being exposed to a normal environment, behaving normally around normal people helps people with cancer feel normal again. At Maggie's, this practice of "normalisation" is evident in several aspects of the programme, from offering to partecipate in physical activities, to inviting people to sit down and sharing stories with others or to quitely isolate themselves with a book, just like at home. It must be said that physical activities such as gentle movement, yoga or Tai chi can be quite difficult for some people, which is why instructors always advise against doing some exercises if they have had a recent operation. What I have observed while participating in this type of activities is that people with cancer often take courses as a way to feel normal again and sometimes even challenge themselves, knowing at the same time that they are in a safe environment.

> Doing a physical activity, yoga or dance or whatever else, may be challenging you physically in ways that you realise are going to be beneficial in the long term. But in that challenge, you know that you're in a safe space because you're in this building and anything happens in this building will be for you, not for somebody else.
>
> (*Move-along_no.2 Barts*)

In this process of normalisation, a feeling of reciprocity prompts visitors to help others by 'giving' rather than 'taking', which is another way to feel rewarded.

> Sometimes I've seen people crying or upset, so I say: 'Would you like a cup of tea?' I'm not a volunteer but I know what it's like to come in and feel sad and uncomfortable and just being offered something by someone it's a peer, in a sense it's a peer exchange, it's a peer kind of support. (…) I remember a bunch of us sat and talked to someone who was worried about radiotherapy and we'd all had radiotherapy and we were trying to comfort her, and I think that's a thing too. Sometimes you feel like you need support and other times you feel like you

can, because you have the energy, give support to other people. And that makes you feel good as well because you think 'okay I've had a shitty experience but at least I can pass on my wisdom to someone else'.

(Follow-up Barts)

By gaining self-confidence, visitors begin to trust others, quickly becoming less concerned about the 'no-confidentiality' of the building, realising that the building is reliable and that it is possible to feel safe even in an open space.

And you see the openness and you think 'oh, there's no confidentiality' here. And I was looking for that, but I could see only those two seats there, by the veranda and, actually, we had a good chat there, totally in the open space, which was nice. It wrapped around you; you could feel safe even in a big space.

(Focus-group_no.2 Dundee)

Knowing that confidentiality is very important in healthcare, and that, surprisingly, Maggie's visitors are relaxed and indifferent to that which is said inside the building that will possibly be carried outside, I asked my participants what was that at Maggie's made them feel this way and what they thought the difference was with NHS confidentiality. The group of women from the art therapy course who participated in a focus group at Maggie's Barts had never thought of this before, and this seemed like a good sign.

I don't know what the difference is, but it's true, I personally don't tell people I go to Maggie's. *I don't know what it is, I think it's so separate from the outside, they are two different worlds.* I think so. I don't know if you've ever been to a festival, I mean for two or three days. You're in a festival away from everything, from another reality, in another world. You never think it works with slightly different rules like leaving your stuff in a tent and you think it will be fine. Nobody will steal anything, and you trust it. You trust the people of that world. *Yes. There's an inherent kindness I think that runs through its core. A kind of school, you, and for yourself and for others, I mean it's really powerful. Yeah, very contagious.*

(Focus-group Barts)

For visitors, entering a Maggie's centre is like stepping into another world that belongs only to them and that they don't want to share outside. At Maggie's, people know that privacy doesn't necessarily mean an enclosed space; on the contrary, thanks to the open space, the sense of trust in others is transmitted from person to person and the whole building is perceived as private and reliable. At this point the visitors, more self-sufficient and able to help others, have entered the third phase of Psychological Flexibility "Doing what matters, acting according to one's value" with trust and respect.

'Making the Biggest Difference' (Affect/Agency) (Visitors' Voice)

Moving from a state of shock to a state of stability, through the stages of adaptation and normalisation, visitors develop affect towards Maggie's. This not only improves the emotional experience—personal and social—that they live, but also the cognitive skills that, thanks to affect, visitors learn to adopt such as planning and decision-making (Iurato, 2020).

> So, I took the courage and came here, and they haven't gotten rid of me since. And I have attended many different courses, such as creative writing, so beautiful.
>
> *(Focus-Group_no.2 Dundee)*

As already confirmed by neuroscience, affect—an *ensemble* in which Spinoza (1632–1677) brings together 'drives, motivations, emotions, and feelings', a central aspect of humanity (Damasio, 2004)—is fundamental for reasoning aimed at decision-making. "Reasoning and decision are so intertwined that they are often used interchangeably and usually imply that the decision maker has a logical strategy" (Damasio, 1994, pp. 165–166). As a matter of fact, at Maggie's people with cancer are able to develop strategies.

> For me, Maggie's is a place where to reground myself away from what's going on out there. If I really want to be recharged, I come here. I know it will never go away. You need strategies to deal with your cancer, you need strategies to deal with the people that surround you when you have cancer, all different kinds of strategy. My strategy to cope is to come to Maggie's.
>
> *(Follow-up Dundee)*

At a neurobiological level, affect leads to the secretion of hormones that improve the body's performance—such as the joy that triggers hunger—also positively influencing the mind in our relationship with the world (Damasio, 2004).

> It can't be disappointing, I'm very aware of my environment when I look around and so the colours, you know, the glass, the coloured glass.
>
> *(Focus-group Barts)*

At this point, Maggie's visitors trust the building and know for sure that the built environment has an impact on them, 'affecting' their perceptual experience (Duncan and Feldman Barrett, 2007).

> Everyone who comes to Maggie's is affected. I'm trying to choose the right word, 'affected by the environment'. And you can compute strengths from the ones affected, and what we can go down lots of different groups. I think every

single person that comes into this building is affected by it, by the building, yes by it.

(Follow-up Dundee)

Perceiving the environment each in their own way, according to the life events that equally 'affected' them, Maggie's visitors learn to evaluate the meaning of these events and process them individually, knowing that the Maggie's centre is always present and reliable.

> No two people's cancer is the same. Everyone's is different. Every experience is different, and we all handle it in different ways. But the Maggie's centre, wherever that centre may be, provides a sanctuary under a therapeutic space with everybody else in it, to have that space, that you can't get anywhere else.
>
> *(Follow-up Dundee)*

Each centre has a different story, which is often very touching due to the commitment behind it. More than anything, though, knowing Maggie Keswick's story helps establish a strong connection to Maggie's philosophy. To this end, in each centre there are always at least two to three copies of Charles Jencks' book *The Architecture of Hope*, which makes staff and visitors feel fuelled with affect and very proud of their centre, while also demonstrating a competitive spirit towards other centres.

> I can't say I would have the same feeling if I went to Kirkcaldy or Edinburgh, because I've never been to any other Maggie's. I think, due to the ethics behind what she [Maggie] was trying to create, getting to know people that have been behind the centre, it helps.
>
> *(Follow-up Dundee)*

Having reached the last stage of the healing process and achieved psychological stability, the old visitors are aware that they must make room for the new ones, knowing that they will come back to to say hello from time to time. There are cases of dependence in which people "cannot do without it" and are unable to detach themselves, to the point that we could define this feeling for Maggie's as an 'affect' that borders on 'love'. Apart from these exceptions, however, visitors are well aware that knowing how to rationally control emotions is extremely important for them to progress.

> Besides architecture that I love, I will be as attached, but it is when that attachment maybe becomes a dependency as well, which I'm wary of, I don't want to be dependent. So, actually leaving here might be quite difficult, if you can't control it. At what point you say 'I'm leaving, Maggie's, now'. Because the philosophy of Maggie's is actually not being dependent, rather it's to move on with your life.
>
> *(Move-along_no.2 Dundee)*

Building and Users: Symbiosis and Shared Mind

Of the four research methods adopted in my ethnographic work—the first two were seen in Chapter 2—the second two consisted of focus groups with visitors and semi-structured interviews with staff, aimed at discovering how the building respectively supports and collaborates with users.

In general, among the visitors and my participants, women were more enthusiastic and less shy than men. For example, during my last week at Maggie's Dundee, when I thought I had already collected enough data from the men's group, a group of women asked me if they could give me their opinion on the building and tell me about their experience. Likewise, at Maggie's Oldham I was quite surprised when on the first day of my fieldwork, the group of women from the Tai chi course asked me to hold a focus group for them. They wanted to know all about my research, and, at the same time, they wanted to let me know their opinion on the architecture of their Maggie's centre. Based on these precedents, as soon as I arrived at Maggie's Barts, I immediately scheduled a focus group and invited the group of women from the art therapy course to participate.

The three focus group discussions touched on many themes, among which *safety*, *normality* and *agency* proved to be the most meaningful, encompassing within the principles of *'feeling at home'*, *'feeling included'* and *'feeling valued'* of Maggie's *Therapeutikos*. The one-to-one interviews with staff members (13 in all) then confirmed that to generate safety, normality and agency in visitors, staff and the building, together, must offer *stimulus, predictability, flexibility*. To learn about all the themes extracted from my ethnographic work in the Maggie's centres, see Frisone (2021). I would like to remind the reader that the ultimate goal of my PhD research was to verify that the work performed 'in tandem' by the building and the staff constituted a 'synergistic power' that generates psychological flexibility in Maggie's visitors.

The most surprising aspect of these group discussions and one-to-one interviews held in the three different Maggie's centres was that, despite the buildings being very distant from each other, not only were the themes that emerged the same, but also the terms used by the participants coincided. For example, in each centre the participants defined the building as 'welcoming', 'calming', 'relaxing', 'safe', 'homely', referring to the Maggie's centre as a 'refuge', 'cocoon', 'sanctuary' or a 'home away from home', which implies the *feeling of being at home*. Or in each centre the participants said that at Maggie's "there is no need to pretend" and that they feel 'themselves' and 'part of the community', meaning that there is a sense of 'normality' and 'identity', which implies the *feeling of being included*. Finally, using terms such as 'openness', 'appreciation' and 'ownership', in each centre the participants meant that in the Maggie's centre they find 'freedom', 'sense of value' and 'agency', which implies the *feeling of being valued*.

This coincidence would have been predictable for the staff receiving the same type of training, and perhaps even for visitors of the same centre taking the same courses, but for me it was incredible to hear the same concepts from three different groups of participants who didn't know each other and lived in different places. But there is more. Besides using the same terms and expressions, what surprised me the most was seeing people behave the same way, especially in the kitchen area or the activity room. Suspecting that there was a 'thread' that connected the buildings making the users speak and act in the same way, I understood that the common denominator resided in the architectural space and, in particular, in one component of it. Adding a piece to Charles Jencks' argument, as we shall see in the next chapter, my finding goes one step further in attributing to the work and spirit of the staff the fact that all centres, however different and wherever located, produce the same psychological effects.

As explained in Chapter 2, while I was looking for a relationship between the architecture and visitors' psychological flexibility that I had discovered in the 'movement', I did not realise, however, that in a Maggie's centre, the open and sensory space triggers another phenomenon that makes the synergy between 'people' and 'place' a 'symbiosis', and between 'people' and 'people' a 'shared mind'. This affective exchange in a "whole realm of human life that is outside consciousness" (Amin and Thrift, 2002, p. 28) is called *empathy*.

Empathy is defined as the involuntary mechanism of "immediate resonance" with the emotions of others, both positive and negative (Boella, 2018). In the healthcare sector, since it was introduced in the nursing sciences in 1973 (Määttä, 2006, cited in Masera, 2007), empathy has been considered a mandatory practice because, in addition to being an integral part of the ethics and philosophy of care, "care without empathy" is considered less effective (Layton, 1979, cited in Masera, 2007*). With Husserl (1982 [1913]), empathy becomes a key concept within the phenomenological method of knowing others. As seen in the introduction, according to the philosopher, the objective external world can only be known in an intersubjective way, and the way in which we relate to others occurs through the *Einfühlung*=in-feeling (=feeling inside) which allows us to relate to others by recognising our living body (*Leib*) as analogous to other bodies moving in space. For Husserl (1982 [1913]), in fact, there can be no perception of the other and it is impossible to live the experience of the other in the first person, without awareness of one's own acting body which cannot be separated from the mechanisms that govern action.

Along these same lines, Husserl's doctoral student Edith Stein built her thesis (later her book) *On the Problem of Empathy* (1916). In addition to confirming her master's ideas on the relationship between the living body and intersubjectivity, Stein (1988 [1917]) had come to understand that *empathy* is the only emotional-cognitive process capable of introducing us to *intersubjectivity* understood as an encounter halfway between two subjects, after one "has realised" or has received the signal that the other is feeling an emotion. Once a subject feels empathy, he/she interrupts the unique experience he/she is having and, through the experience of 'otherness', recreates a new one with the other subject. In this round-trip work between the two subjects, mutual knowledge does not grow through similarity but through difference, that is, for what they are not or what they have not yet lived, becoming an element of the most intimate experience, that of the "feel together" (Boella and Buttarelli, 2000 from).

However, for phenomenologists, *empathy* is not a feeling of participation or sharing, but the direct experience of the existence of others who move in the world, experience emotions and have autonomous intentions. In short, it is the *discovery of the other* in our way of living the intersubjective nature of the human condition (Boella, 2018).

> Discovering the other means removing it from the anonymous mass (…) and restoring its singularity. This is the only possible beginning of hospitality and welcome.
>
> (Boella, 2018, p. 14*)

In a Maggie's centre, thanks to the openness of the space, people can observe each other and, while gaining confidence, think: "if others do it, I can do it, too", feeling reassured that "I am not the only one" (Howells, 2016, 8:53). Under the lens of Neuroscience, through empathy, the relationship with the 'other' is a relation of similarity ('they are just like me') of which an important component is the common experience of action (sharing at the kitchen table). This relationship of similarity is generated by the "as if" mechanism of *embodied simulation* (ES) theorised by Vittorio Gallese (2009), the neuroscientist we met in Chapter 2 who, in the 1990s, as part of Rizzolatti's group, discovered mirror neurons also in humans. Seen as neural correlates of 'intercorporeality'—i.e. a bodily openness to others—or *embodied simulation,* mirror neurons are the primary means of knowing others (Gallese, 2013*). As mentioned, by far anticipating these discoveries, Merleau-Ponty had intuited that the intersubjectivity of the observer and the observed could only be resolved if the intention-movement link was analysed: from the movement of the other, one perceives the intention that generated the movement itself (Di Fazio, 2015). In addition to triggering motor equivalence in the process of 'perception and action' explained in Chapter 2, in fact, the neural mechanism of motor simulation activates the interchangeability of points of view and makes us understand the feelings and mental states of others, seeing or hearing what the other sees or hears. In short, mirror neurons are the biological proof of empathy which is the fundamental condition of intersubjective relationships (Di Fazio, 2015).

> Intersubjectivity is based on an 'undifferentiated awareness' of the action through which two individuals emerge as similar and separate beings at the same time.
>
> (Gallese, 2009, cited in Mezzalira, 2019, pp. 56–57*)

But while phenomenology fails to explain how this awareness develops naturally, the discovery of mirror neurons succeeds (Gallagher and Meltzoff, 1996 cited by Mezzalira, 2019).

> The discovery of mirror neurons offers an empirical edge to the conception of intersubjectivity seen as reciprocity and correlation between the self which another self that is simultaneously, in many ways and first and foremost, another myself"
>
> (Gallese, 2009, p. 15*)

Although Edith Stein, after her conversion to Catholicism in 1922, devoted herself to the elaboration of a 'theory of the person', and despite the image of the human being that arises from Husserl's thought, especially if reread in the light of the discoveries of neuroscience, is current and urgent (Gallese, 2009*), the phenomenological thinking on empathy has not left a complete theory behind. This means that today empathy should no longer be seen in a theoretical framework, but in a practical application (Boella, 2018). In this, while the neurobiological imaging aimed at emphasising empathy progresses in the laboratory, at Maggie's, within the design principle of 'spatial interaction rather than walls', empathy is enacted every day as a "resource for practicing humanity" (Boella, 2021*). By getting involved, discovering the other "for better or for worse", becoming curious to know more—where *curious* from the Latin term *curiosus* (=who takes care of) finds its root in *cura* (=care)— staff and visitors, who did not know each other until recently, suddenly enter into a relationship of intimacy which "widens" or "tightens" (Boella, 2021*). And when the empathy of the staff merges with that of the built environment, visitors can experience something very special.

> One of the things that people say about the Maggie's centre is that there is empathy in the building, and when it meets the empathy of the staff then this incredible emotional chain reaction can happen. Something that is extraordinary entitled to the person, because they can generally turn towards reality, whatever stand they want.
>
> (Howells, 2016, 14:28)

What Buildings Do to People

To recognise the therapeutic nature of an architecture or, in more phenomenological terms, to understand its experiential dimension, I introduce here the theme of the 'push' that buildings give in shaping the practices of those who use them (Kraftl and Adey 2008, p. 219).

The idea that buildings can 'act' on us and 'push' our bodies into space was highlighted by Thomas Gieryn in his article *What buildings do* (2002). where he confirmed that, buildings are evolving projects, in a constant process of making and re-making (Ingold, 2013) and as such we should move away from and look beyond static notions of artefacts that appear to be compartmentalised in their final stages. According to Gieryn, buildings can do many things—contain, hide, represent, entertain, prevent and much more—but above all they stabilise social life, giving solidity, identity, and durability to society against the forces of change. With all their imperfections, "buildings don't just sit and impose themselves" (Gieryn 2002, p. 1), rather they interact. Buildings live thanks to the people who use them and associate meanings with them; in exchange the buildings protect, support and arouse feelings and emotions.

During my interviews with Maggie's staff, I discovered that when the building is still under construction, Maggie's adopts the intermediate solution of "Maggie's Interim", welcoming visitors to mobile homes whose interior closely resembles a Maggie's centre, obtaining excellent results. This discovery raised in me the great dilemma of whether, for the purpose of Maggie's mission, sophisticated and unconventional architecture is really essential to provide psychological support and, in general, to create a therapeutic environment. Indeed, the data showed that the absence of the building did not affect the work of the staff that much. At the same time, the presence of the building which, as seen, invites visitors to linger longer in the open space, helping them to prepare for the meeting with the psychologists and convincing them to return the next time, demonstrates that the mere support given by the staff, however valuable, is not enough. During the COVID-19 pandemic (2019–2022), Maggie's then strengthened the third support option 'Maggie's Online' as the only form of assistance and attendance was still very high. At that point the question that arose was: how much does the environment matter and do people matter?

Contrary to what I expected, Sabina Brennan (2015)—the psychologist from Trinity College Dublin whom we met in chapters 3 and 4—said that if we are fully present in the 'moment', living life and having a very full experience, sometimes, the environment or the building that we are in does not matter.

> Okay, I hate to say that to an architect, your mind isn't anywhere else. It's just in that moment, pick whatever from from your life and sometimes, even if it's an awful surrounding, that doesn't matter because it's the living that matters.
>
> (Brennan, 2015, 42:58)

Of the same opinion was a visitor, a former nurse, who argued that if you choose to work in the clinical setting what matters is assisting people regardless of the surrounding conditions.

> I was a nurse, and you go into it because that's what you want to do, you want to help people. So, I don't think that the building will make it different, maybe it makes it pleasant to both the staff and the people who attend. I think also that there's an ethos here. That is, maybe, very helpful to them to carry out certain helpful tools to the staff. But it doesn't matter. If you are in a war area, and you're a nurse, you go and you help, do what you can for the patient, you do the same job under different circumstances. But the conditions, the spatial conditions are not there to help you.
>
> (*Focus-group_no.2 Dundee*)

Finally, even Maggie's psychologists, while confirming that the building is "with them" in accompanying visitors during their healing process, felt compelled to say that they hoped to have been helpful with their 'therapies' regardless of the presence of the building.

> Have I been helpful to people, when I've worked in an NHS room? I hope so, I don't think they've had a different psychologist. I think this helps, and I think

this is nice for me and it's nice for them. And this is ideal that this is the therapy that people get, whether it's here or whether it's at the NHS; I hope it wouldn't impact on the work I do. But it just makes sense if you're in a nicer space and, you know, we are here and it's a nice place, it puts people at ease, it is going to be hopefully helpful for the work we're going to do. It's hard to tell if I can see the difference, because I should take the same person to two different places. But this is nicer, it's more therapeutic.

(Psychologist Oldham)

As mentioned, perceived in different ways depending on people's background and life aspirations, the physical environment may or may not count depending on the circumstances, and, if it counts, it will certainly have a different meaning for each of us. Overall, all in agreement that "it makes sense to have it" if the environment is more 'pleasant' or more 'therapeutic', but also that we are all different 'individuals' for whom every day is different, knowing the openness of the Maggie's centre—a menu of spaces—perhaps, the answer to my question is simply that the building matters to the extent that it is deliberately left open to any interpretation so that each of us can 'see' whatever we want.

When I arrived at Maggie's Dundee, I didn't even see the building. I didn't see the architecture. For me it was just my problem and the people standing in front of me there to help me; only later, I understood what the building was like.

(Focus-group_no.1 Dundee)

Anyone who thinks that the environment is important is convinced that people count too, indeed that both count.

Often people might see it's not about the building, it's about what happens in the building and people in the building. I think it's both actually, I think we could have a beautiful building which would do an awful lot anyway. But I think the right people are important. I think there is something, I can't explain it, but there is something about having a conversation in this building, which is different from having that even in another nice building, not necessarily in a dark space, but I think there's something very unique about this building. I think it allows you to pause or even allows you to stop talking and look at something and think. Whatever I'm doing, whatever the visual is doing to our brains is soothing and comforting. I think this building is quite special, but I don't know if it's because we love it so much.

(CCS_no.2 Dundee)

Through their eyes, Maggie's staff can see the ongoing dialogue between the visitors and the building and feel that the architecture unites them: offering *stimulus*, *flexibility*, *predictability* the building generates surprise and wonder.

It would be beauty. I'm not sure if that's quite the right word, but there's something about, when people are sitting in this space, in this building, something is generating in them, despite their illness, they get in touch with the feeling of safety, the feeling of space, art, there is this sort of stimulus there, and there are different kinds of stimuli given the fact that we have different kinds of art, the furniture, the soft furnishings.

(*Psychologist Dundee*)

If buildings 'act' and 'push' only in the presence of people, just as their therapeutic action is achieved only if people use them and interact with them, ultimately, we can say that it is the ability of architecture to establish a dialogue with individuals that makes us indentity the therapeutic nature of a building or, in more phenomenological terms, its experiential dimension. As we will see in Chapter 7, confirming the contradictory nature of a therapeutic environment, its effectiveness will no longer be based on its typology or function, but rather on the emotions and feelings it transmits to us, leading us to recognise it as an architecture that makes us feel good.

References

Amin, A. and Thrift, N. (2002) *Cities: Reimagining the Urban*. Cambridge, UK: Polity Press

Aristotle (350 BC) *Metaphysics*, Book 8, part 6. transl. by Ross, W.D. (1924) in Stevenson, D.C., Web Atomics (1994–2000). http://classics.mit.edu//Aristotle/metaphysics.html

Boella, L. (2018) *Empatie. L'esperienza empatica nella società del conflitto*. Milan: Cortina Editore

Boella, L. (2021) 'L'empatia, risorsa in un mondo in crisi'. https://www.youtube.com/watch?v=NpZPVIbxTNM&ab_channel=AssoCounseling

Boella, L. and Buttarelli, A. (2000) *Per amore di altro. L'Empatia a partire da Edith Stein*. Milan: Cortina Editore

Bratton, J., Mills, J. H., Pyrch, T. and Sawchuk, P. (2008) *Workplace Learning: A Critical Introduction*. Ontario and New York: Higher Education University of Toronto Press

Brennan, S. (2015) 'Patterns of Neurons Firing'. Interview with Sabina Brennan. Interviewed by N. McLaughlin and Y. Manolopoulou for Losing Myself. http://www.losing-myself.ie/pages/patterns-neurons-firing/

Butterfield, A. and Martin, D. (2016) 'Affective Sanctuaries: Understanding Maggie's as Therapeutic Landscapes', *Landscape Research*, 41(6), pp. 695–706

Cambridge Dictionary (2023) "Definition of Synergy". https://dictionary.cambridge.org/dictionary/english/synergy

Chalmers, A. (1826) *The Whole Works of the Right Rev. Edward Reynolds, Lord Bishop of Norwich*, Volume 2. London: Holdsworth

Damasio, A. (1994). *Descartes' Error: Emotion, Reason, and the Human Brain*. London: Vintage

Damasio, A. (2004) *Looking for Spinoza. Joy, Sorrow and the Feeling Brain*. London: Vintage

D'Avenia, A. (2018) '15. Piccola Filosofia per matti', *Corriere della Sera*, 7 May. https://www.corriere.it/alessandro-davenia-letti-da-rifare/18_maggio_06/15-piccola-filosofia-matti-alessandro-d-avenia-letti-da-rifare-f0c88e92-5130-11e8-b393-1dfa8344f8a7.shtml

Di Fazio, C. (2015) 'The Free Body. Notes on Maurice Merleau-Ponty's Phenomenology of Movement', *SIF-Praha.Cz*. https://www.sif-praha.cz/wp-content/uploads/2013/04/The-free-body.pdf

Duncan, S. and Feldman Barrett, L. (2007) 'Affect Is a Form of Cognition: A Neurobiological Analysis', *Cognition and Emotion*, 21(6), pp. 1184–1211

Frisone, C. (2021) *The Role of Architecture in the Therapeutic Environment. The Case Study of the Maggie's Cancer Care Centre*, Doctoral Thesis, School of Architecture, Faculty of TDE, Oxford Brookes University. https://doi.org/10.24384/0ejy-7815

Gallese, V. (2009). 'Neuroscienze e fenomenologia', *Treccani Terzo Millennio*, I, pp. 1–32. https://www.treccani.it/enciclopedia/neuroscienze-e-fenomenologia_%28XXI-Secolo%29/

Gallese, V. (2013) 'Corpo non mente. Le neuroscienze cognitive e la genesi di soggettività ed intersoggettività', *Educazione Sentimentale*, 20, pp. 8–24

Gepshtein, S. and Berger, T. (2020) *Dynamics of Architectural Experience in the Perceptual Field*. 16 January. https://www.youtube.com/watch?v=HI7s8OhZpT4&ab_channel=AMPS

Gieryn, T. (2002) 'What Buildings Do', *Theory and Society*, 31, pp. 35–74

Harris, R. (2009) *ACT Made Simple: An Easy-To-Read Primer on Acceptance and Commitment Therapy*. Oakland, CA: New Harbinger Publications

Harris, R. (2013) *Getting Unstuck in ACT: A Clinician's Guide to Overcoming Common Obstacles in Acceptance and Commitment Therapy*. Oakland, CA: New Harbinger Publications

Hayes, S.C.(2017)*Psychological Flexibility: How Love Turns Pain into Purpose*.11 May. https://www.youtube.com/watch?v=W3NmN1F_M1I&ab_channel=FamilyActionNetwork

Hayes, S. C. (2021) *ACT*. https://contextualscience.org/act

Hayes, S. C. and Smith, S. (2005) *Get Out of Your Mind and Into Your Life. The New Acceptance & Commitment Therapy*. Oakland, CA: New Harbinger Publications

Heidegger, M. (1971 [1954]) 'Building, Dwelling, Thinking', in Hofstadter, A. (ed. and transl.) *Poetry, Language, Thought*. New York: Harper Colophon Books, pp. 1–9

Howells, L. (2016) 'Synergy between People and Place', *TEDxTalks*. https://www.youtube.com/watch?v=tvE78D30CbQ

Husserl, E. (1982 [1913]) *Ideas Pertaining to a Pure Phenomenology and to a Phenomenological Philosophy. Volume II, First Book: General Introduction to a Pure Phenomenology*. Translated by F. Kersten. The Hague: Nijhoff

Ingold, T. (2013) *Making: Anthropology, Archaeology, Art and Architecture*. London and New York: Routledge.

Ingold, T. (2013) *Making: Anthropology, Archaeology, Art and Architecture*. London and New York: Routledge.

Iurato, G. (2020) 'Affettività e cognizione: una breve sinossi storico-bibliografica', *HAL*, Id: hal-02568824. https://hal.archives-ouvertes.fr/hal-02568824/document

Jacobs, J. (2006) 'A Geography of Big Things', *Cultural Geographies*, 13, pp. 1–27

Jencks, C. (2017). 'Maggie's Architecture: The Deep Affinities Between Architecture and Health', *Architectural Design*, 87, p. 2.

Kashdan, T. and Rottenberg, J. (2010) 'Psychological Flexibility as a Fundamental Aspect of Health', *Clinical Psychology Review* 30, pp. 865–878

Koffka, K. (1935) *Principles of Gestalt Psychology*. London: Lund Humphries

Kraftl, P. and Adey, P. (2008) 'Architecture/Affect/Inhabitation: Geographies of Being-in Buildings', *Annals of the Association of American Geographers*, 98, pp. 213–231

Mallgrave H.F. (2013) *Architecture and Embodiment. The Implications of the New Sciences and Humanities for Design*. London and New York: Routledge

Martin, D. (2014). 'The Choreography of The Kitchen Table: The Agency of Everyday Spaces in the Experience of Care'. *Psycho-Oncology*, 23, pp. 203–204

Martin, D. (2016) 'Curating Space, Choreographing Care: The Efficacy of the Everyday', in Bates, C., Imrie, R. and Kullman, K. (eds.) *Care and Design: Bodies, Buildings, Cities*. Oxford: Wiley, pp. 39–57

Martin, D. (2020) 'Between Bodies and Buildings: The Place of Comfort within Therapeutic Spaces', in Crang, P., Mcnally, D. and Price, L. (eds.) *Geographies of Comfort*. London: Ashgate/Routledge, chap. 14

Martin, D., Nettleton, S. and Buse, C. (2019) 'Affecting Care: Maggie's Centres and the Orchestration of Architectural Atmospheres', *Social Science & Medicine*, 240, pp. 1–8

Masera, G. (2007) 'L'empatia in Edith Stein: la giusta distanza per essere accanto all'altro', I Luoghi della Cura Rivista Online. https://www.luoghicura.it/operatori/professioni/2007/09/lempatia-edith-stein-la-giusta-distanza-accanto-allaltro/

Merleau-Ponty, M. (1963 [1942]) *The Structure of Behaviour*. Trans. Fisher, A. L. Boston [MA]: Beacon

Mezzalira, S. (2019). Neuroscienze e fenomenologia. Il caso dei 'neuroni specchio'. Padova: University Press

Relph, E. (1976) *Place and Placelessness*. London: Pion

Seamon, D. and Mugerauer, R. (1985) *Dwelling, Place and Environment. Toward a Phenomenology of Person and World*. Dordrecht: Nijhof

Stein, E. (1988 [1917]) *On the Problem of Empathy,* trans. en.1964. Norwell, MA: Kluwer Academic Publishers

von Uexküll, J. (1926) *Theoretical Biology*. New York: Harcourt, Brace & Co.

Wild, J. (1962) 'Foreword', in Merleau-Ponty, M. (1963 [1942]) *The Structure of Behaviour*. Trans. Fisher, A. L. Boston [MA]: Beacon, p. xiii

Wolinsky, H. (2019) 'I Have Cancer. Please Don't Call Me a 'Survivor'', *MedPage Today*, 15 April. https://www.medpagetoday.com/special-reports/apatientsjourney/79229

Wright, D., Corner, J., Hopkinson, J. and Foster, C. (2006) 'Listening to the Views of People Affected by Cancer about Cancer Research: An Example of Participatory Research in Setting the Cancer Research Agenda', *Health Expect,* 9(1), pp. 3–12

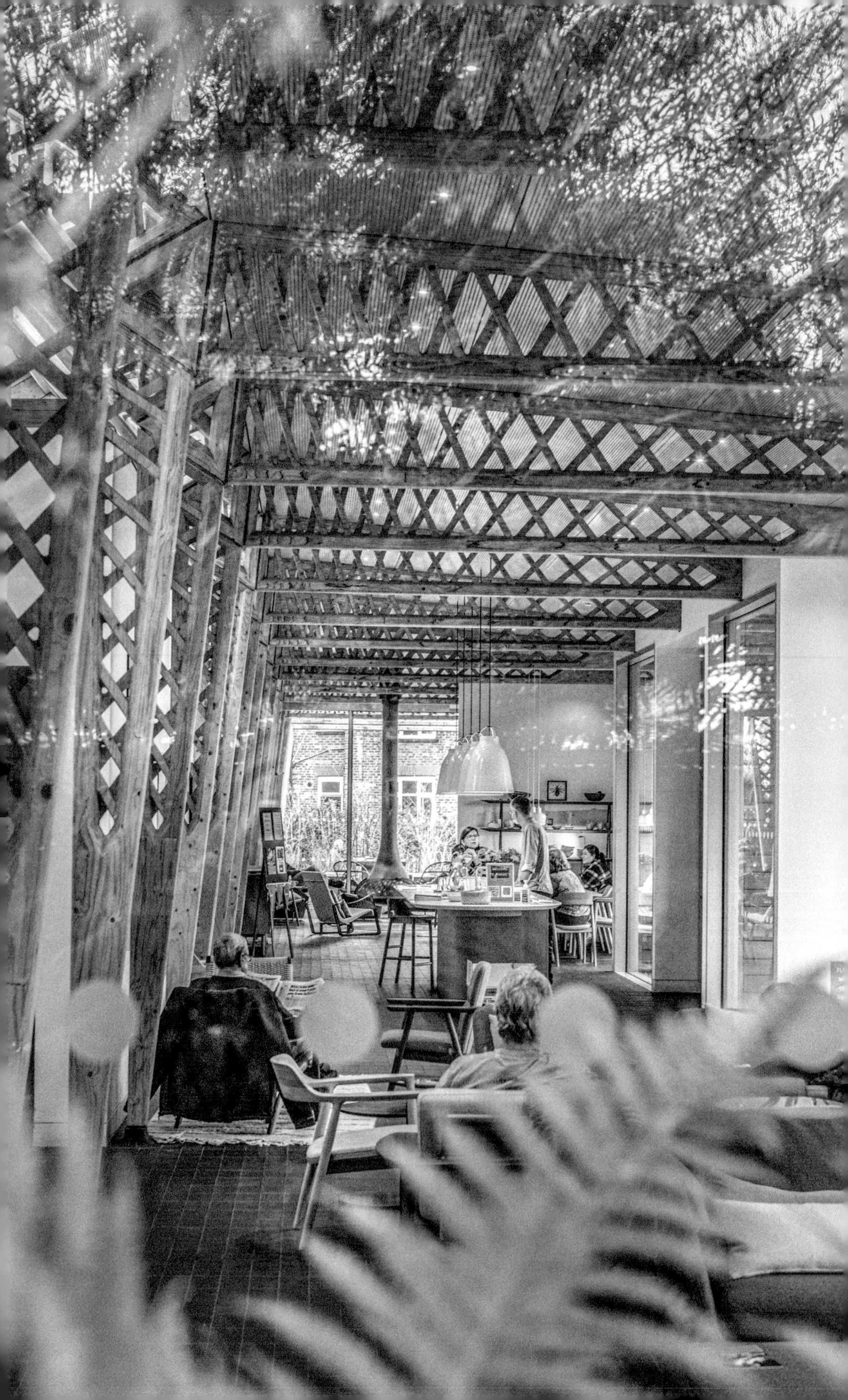

6

MAGGIE'S PHENOMENOLOGY

A Phenomenological Synergy

At the still point of the turning world. Neither flesh nor fleshless;
Neither from nor towards; at the still point, there the dance is,
But neither arrest nor movement. And do not call it fixity,
Where past and future are gathered. Neither movement from nor towards,
Neither ascent nor decline. Except for the point, the still point,
There would be no dance, and there is only the dance.

T.S Eliot, Burnt Norton, Four Quartets, 1936

As Lesley Howells explains, while performing T.S. Eliot's quartet *At the still point of the turning world* (Burnt Norton, Four Quartets, 1936) in her TedxDundee Talk (2016), it is the synergy between the bespoke architecture of the Maggie's centre combined in a vibrant 'fluid dance' with the people within that enables and creates the concept of psychological flexibility. By creating a 'vicinity' between people and the surrounding spatial field, the synergy allows Maggie's visitors to be present and open to reality. As mentioned, this means that people open up to the concept of not fighting, finding freedom in the choice that is offered to them. And this is encouraged by Maggie's *Therapeutikós*—i.e. the compassionate and caring attitude of the *people* combined with the unconventional architecture of the *place*—which invites visitors to participate in suffering, giving birth, as it was in ancient Greece, to a therapeutic environment. On the one hand, Maggie's asks visitors to live with impermanence, that is, with the sense of the unknown about the future; on the other hand, compensating for this uncertainty, it offers them human support which, thanks to the building and the 'openness' of the space, with solidarity, for "better or for worse" and in "being close", generates a "therapeutic empathy",

DOI: 10.4324/9781003244516-6

also thanks to the fact that suffering is, unfortunately, still today, the privileged way to shake us from our isolation and become aware of the existence of the other (Boella, 2021).

Building on the participants' insights outlined in Chapter 5 and the uncertainty of their "I don't know what it is," "I don't know how to explain it"—which made me intuit that phenomenology had something to do with it—, in attempting to decode the therapeutic process, I needed to understand the true nature of the synergy advanced by Lesley Howells and unravel the phenomenological essence of Maggie's space. By interviewing Maggie's psychologists, I had discovered that the feelings of agency and mastery that are evidently elicited in visitors certainly stem from the stimulating physical space enhanced by the warm atmosphere, but only in combination with an apparently informal way of conversing, a more subconscious way the staff frame conversations and interactions, which is critical to visitors. By telling them it's okay to be emotional and encouraging them to act normally and walk freely around the building, people take the lead. In fact, even in the absence of staff, a strong sense of agency is activated in people because they know that the building, seen as an 'active agent' rather than a 'passive context' (Hensel, 2010), can replace the staff at any time in helping visitors access the 'many things' Maggie's offers them.

As we know, the 'many things'—i.e. the multifaceted reality of the Maggie's centre derived from the "thousand crazy ideas" (*Murphy, 06.11.2018*) that Maggie wanted to offer to people with cancer—led Jencks to identify the centre as 'hybrid', endowed with a real power. The hybrid, the 'whole' or the synergistic coexistence of 'many things', recalls the Gestalt motto "the whole is more than the sum of its parts" (Koffka, 1935, p. 176), which is ultimately the unallocated definition of synergy and that which Merleau-Ponty identifies in his concept of 'structure'. To explain what 'structure' or rather the "spatial structure within the visual field" is, in his first book *The Structure of Behaviour* (1963 [1942]), Merleau-Ponty compares space to a football field that "is pervaded with lines of force (the 'yard lines'; those which demarcate the 'penalty area') and articulated in sectors" which will offer opportunities for action "as if the player were unaware of it". Thus, the field becomes a 'structured arena' and "the player becomes one with it and feels the direction of the goal" (1963 [1942], p. 168).

With the expression "becomes one with it"—somehow inherent in the concept of *Umwelt*—I clarify here the concept of 'embodied experience' already mentioned earlier in this book. For Merleau Ponty (1963 [1942]), not only does the spatial structure of the field release forces that move and guide the player, but, in turn, the player will act on it, modifying the space which will change due to the movement of the body. It is in this dialectical exchange between player and field, between man and the world, that the two merge in a space enveloping "as in a garment" (Vischer, 1873, quoted in Mallgrave, 2013, p. 122). The terms often used by Maggie's users, 'atmosphere', 'aura', 'ambience', recall an 'enveloping feeling' generated by forces acting on the body and, therefore, on the brain, which processes the experience as an embodied perception of space that becomes difficult to describe ("I don't know how to explain it", "I don't know what it is").

As Merleau-Ponty suggests, it is only through 'habit' that we acquire the ability to 'in-habit' the space, since familiarity makes it easy for us to navigate. However, at the level of sensory perception, familiarity is the body's ability to dampen responses to a continuous stimulus, causing us to gradually lose attention and ignore details (or exclude distractions such as noise) (Hale, 2017); that is why every act of focusing must be renewed (Merleau-Ponty 2012 [1945], p. 249). Being in synergy with the place or 'structure', Maggie's visitors are continually stimulated to move and to understand the intentionality of others. If it is true that my ethnographic work proved that phenomenology—which in its methodological principle is an investigation of correlations (Held, 2003)—was the correct methodology to adopt in my research, it also revealed that the synergy between people and place that the Maggie's centre creates is a phenomenological synergy an indispensable condition for triggering the process of psychological flexibility. In this story of mine, I bring evidence that, together with the stimulating social context that aspires to 'spatial interaction rather than walls', the 'spatial structure' is what enables the phenomenal field or experiential field.

Today is a beautiful day, the kitchen is quiet and sunny. After sitting down at the kitchen table and taking some notes, I decide to move to the oval counter to introduce myself and my research to a woman who is there reading a newspaper. Philly is happy to meet me and speak with me. After listening briefly to her, I understand that she is an out-of-the-ordinary woman, for several reasons. First, a long time ago, she refused treatment for her first bout of breast cancer and managed to treat herself with alternative methods. Because she had refused chemical treatment and was 'different' from everyone else, although she liked the building, she was one of the few Maggie's visitors who did not like coming to Maggie's. She felt like she did not fit in, so she walked away. But in the winter 2018 the cancer came back and she was close to dying. So, she decided to accept the traditional protocol and return to Maggie's where this time she felt like 'one of them'.

Totally taken by these stories and fascinated by the way she is telling them, I haven't noticed that, in the meantime, 3 or 4 other people are sitting at the oval counter with us, chatting, and the kitchen has filled up with people, scattered in various groups conversing. One of the volunteers goes around the groups to collect empty tea cups and serve new ones. While all of this is happening, totally engrossed in Philly's story, filled with grief and anger at the hardships she's encountered, unable to contain them, I find myself in tears. The volunteer immediately comes over to offer her help, but it is enough for her and all the people around us to smile at me for things to go back to normal right away.

(Fieldnotes Dundee, 17.09.2019, 7:30 pm)

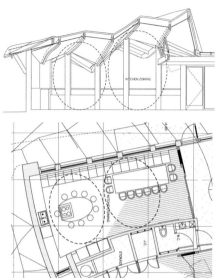
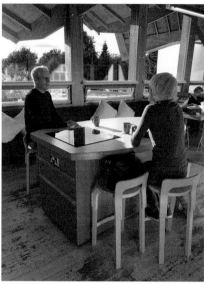

FIGURE 6.1A–6.1C Maggie's Dundee (2003), plan and section diagrammes of the 'hidden' structure of the experiential field. View of the oval counter wrapped in an imaginary 'bubble' of privacy enclosed underneath the intricate trussed ceiling (Drawings courtesy of Frank Gehry with diagramme by the author) (©Courtesy of Maggie's).

One aspect of the building's 'magic' (Howells, 2017) has actually just happened and revealed itself. Testing this experience first-hand with my body and mind, I cried unreservedly despite the surrounding crowds. The spatial structure, which divides the open kitchen into sub-areas each contained under the many intricate trusses, had provided 'bubbles' of privacy that isolated Philly and me from everyone; at the same time, the open visual field had allowed other people to see me and encourage me in the moment of crisis, giving me the strength to regain control. By allowing empathy and intersubjectivity, the spatial structure supports people by isolating them from other conversations, yet uniting them through voices, sounds, movements and smiles. In the experiential field intimacy and openness can coexist (Figure 6.1A–6.1C).

After being defined as a 'vicinity' between people and place through 'spatial interaction rather than walls'—guided by the 'structure' or 'totality' of the open space in which people with cancer are called to act freely and access the 'many things' that the hybrid space of the Maggie's centre represents—, revealing itself as a 'fusion' of people immersed in the experiential field, Maggie's synergy between people and place becomes a 'phenomenological synergy', the connection between 'body' and 'space'. Seeing synergy in the context of phenomenology will confirm us that architectural space is not empty but full of forces that move people through continuous stimulation from the experiential field and will explain the therapeutic process that connects cancer reality, experiential field and psychological flexibility.

Body and Space: Premise to the Therapeutic Process

During my ethnographic work, my bodily presence in the three centres was certainly an alien element, because of my role as a researcher as well as because of my physical presence. However, my participation in the centre's activities served to take the pressure off both myself and the visitors, except on one occasion during my first week at Maggie's Dundee. We had just started the focus group with the men's group, when a visitor blurted out blaming me for only being there "just to look at the architecture and not to understand the real content (i.e. cancer)" (*Focus group 2_Dundee*). I tried to explain that, in truth, my work aimed at incorporating me into Maggie's environment, and becoming a temporary member of the community, so as to understand from the inside what was in the building that made people feel good. Yet, the more I talked the more I realised that my interlocutor and I were talking about two different things. Only when I told him about my brother's experience with brain cancer, which lasted almost two years in distressing conditions, did the visitor change his attitude and accept my presence and myself as 'one of them'. At Maggie's, it is not enough to be part of the space, you have to be part of the community.

In a Maggie's centre, the person's body blends naturally and harmoniously with the surrounding space and, as seen, is constantly urged to move through various modalities including physical activities such as gentle movement, yoga and Tai chi, which is a Chinese practice—one of the 'many things' Maggie wanted to offer people from the start—based on physical exercise whose movements express what is inside someone's (mind). Being physical (body and breath), and not meditative (soul), the concentration goes to the body which, moving as though it were a fluid, resembles a dance even if, in reality, Tai chi is a martial art. The mind, at the centre, controls movement and balance. In my notes, I wrote:

> You never stop, even within a single movement, hands, arms and body move making curves and circles almost like a long ribbon could move in the wind. This magic movement sets the body in the centre, like a point, around which all the fluids (limbs) spin. The light is suspended, and it helps to reveal the structural ceiling. All the exercises refer to objects (ball), nature (horizon), or universe (stars, sky, moon). It is like bringing sky and horizon within us. Everything starts from Tai chi.
>
> (*Fieldnotes Dundee, 23.09.2019, 7:15 pm*)

Physical activity and body movement are essential in distracting from stressful or depressive situations. As seen in the previous chapter, referring to the body as something that we carry with us—i.e. a welcoming home that we refer to during times of crisis and use as a means to create comforting places in the surrounding space—body and space are necessary to establish deep relationships with others (D'Avenia, 2018), which is the premise for generating a therapeutic process.

We know from Merleau-Ponty that the body is the key means to learning in human experience. From this point of view, the model of the living body (*Leib*) as something *dependent on* and, at the same time, *inseparable from* its environment—"one's own body is in the world just as the heart is in the organism: it continuously breathes life into the visible spectacle, animates it and nourishes it from within, and forms a system with it" (2012 [1945], p. 209)—is what allows an individual to become part of the world and being, in turn, its projection: "and the subject is inseparable from the world, but from a world that it itself projects" (Merleau-Ponty 2012 [1945], p. 454). These concepts of the body as inseparable from and the projection of its environment—once again our *Umwelt*—are ultimately what helped me to put myself in the 'shoes' of Maggie's users and to understand that, once immersed in space, the skin of the body is the only limit between us and the world, which is nothing but a continuation of us (Merleau-Ponty, 2012 [1945]).

Embodying the Cancer Reality

But what is it exactly that connects body and space? Maggie's community shares a common trait—cancer—and thanks to the particular architecture and professional support of the staff, people are in control. The staff says that old visitors "almost erase it" and cancer is no longer a topic of conversation. And because they no longer need to talk about their cancer, even though they still have it, people can actually start talking about something else.

> Ironically, over time, the conversation about cancer becomes less and less frequent and, in this sense, Maggie's is a therapeutic space. To some extent it removes that, and it is a really important part of helping people normalise what's going on in them.
> (*Centre Head Royal Marsden, 14.02.2020*)

Although there are days at Maggie's when you see people who are tired, forgetting that their life expectancy is short, it's quite common to enter the building and, thanks to the cheery atmosphere which distracts from their illness, not being able to distinguish visitors who are sick from those who are well. As described in Chapter 5, this derives from the constant invitation addressed to people with cancer to act normally. In this normalisation practice, as already seen in Chapter 3, the kitchen table is an essential tool to start the day, representing the visitors' travel companion from day one by encouraging people to sit around it and start talking.

Recalling Jencks' philosophy of 'kitchenism', which expresses colloquiality and good humour, around the kitchen table visitors can have different types of conversations, in small groups, in large groups or just with the staff. At the same table, there are also visitors who sit in silence and listen to the others, and who suddenly, one day, open up and start talking. "When you have cancer, you don't want to be part of the group, quite the contrary" (*Murphy, 06.11.2018*). Indeed, what is very difficult with cancer is the sense of isolation, even though people often choose to isolate themselves to feel protected. Among the privacy control mechanisms, 'personal space'—which is the invisible boundary surrounding the *self*—serves to safeguard one's sense of identity and is crucial for the individual to be in balance with the environment (Hall, 1966). Although asocial, single visitors like to be present, in eye and sonar contact with the others, watching and listening. Free to isolate themselves, what counts at Maggie's is that they never feel 'alone'.

Along the journey with cancer, from diagnosis to recovery, from crisis to recuperation (De Botton, 2023)—which luckily still happens—the building accompanies visitors by offering its spaces and all the conditions of warmth and peace necessary for people to identify the Maggie's centre with a 'hug', a metaphor often used also to define the staff. When people cry—because "here it is okay to cry"—Maggie's brings back memories of times when emotions were allowed. And since the Maggie's centre is not the place where people with cancer receive the bad news, but, rather, the place where they can recover from it or even share the good news with great participation from all, alongside the crying, we can witness the complete opposite emotion of joy. At Maggie's, hearing a great deal of laughter is common and older visitors are not ashamed to laugh in the presence of newcomers in tears, because they know that very soon, the new visitors will be in the same position as them. Within this ambivalent scene, the open space allows people to witness all kinds of emotions and actions which, through empathy, will activate a chain of positive reactions; from a neuroscientific perspective, mirror neurons discharge, people start imitating themselves and the psychological healing process begins (Figure 6.2).

Seeing the other visitors laughing, the people who had been crying up to that moment react by stopping crying and start smiling, as well as observing the staff busy in the kitchen, newcomers feel encouraged to help; or visitors interested in

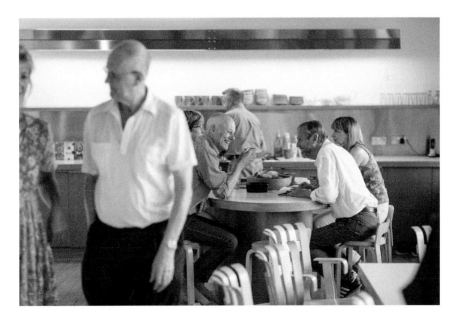

FIGURE 6.2   At Maggie's, hearing laughter is common and older visitors are not ashamed to laugh in the presence of newcomers in tears (Maggie's Dundee, 2003) (Courtesy of Maggie's).

participating in a group activity but are too shy to try, will be able to do it the next time. This unassuming but psychologically sophisticated way of interacting solidly between staff and old visitors that benefits newcomers is, as we now know, facilitated by the openness and flexibility of the building, which is ultimately what connects people and place, body and space. As Laura Lee says: "One of the things that architecture has been able to offer at Maggie's is providing a unique way of helping people relate to each other" (Lee@*V&A Dundee, 2019*).

When undergoing radiation treatments, visitors go to the hospital every day for four to five weeks, for a total of 25 treatments, and often stop by Maggie's before returning home. Many people say that "the reason I do this is because it bridges the gap between the clinic and home". Sitting in a quiet space while having a hot drink contemplating what is happening to them, visitors can rid themselves of clinical stress out, and ponder the idea that once they leave, they will feel better. For people with cancer, the Maggie's centre represents the interface between home and hospital, 'the space between' where they can stop and recharge or reflect to find the very essence of who they are when everything around them is falling to pieces. Using the quote attributed to Viktor Frankl (1905–1997), which says that we cannot control what is happening to us in life, and that the only space we can control is our mind and how we respond to it, Maggie's psychologists invite visitors to not struggle against it but rather to turn towards reality.

> Between stimulus and response there is a space. In that space is our power to choose our response. In our response lies our freedom and growth.
>
> (Viktor Frankl, quoted in Covey, 1989, p. 70)

Effectively, between the trigger and the response, the Maggie's centre is a 'still point', a free, open, flexible and reliable space to be interpreted and taken in a different way by each of us.

Maggie's Experiential Field

The link between our body and the surrounding space is a tenacious one: if the external environment influences and induces the movements of our body, it is equally true that the action of our body affects the surrounding environment. In this process of interaction with the place, the body imposes its habits as well as grasping the challenges of the context. At Maggie's what enhances this link by transforming the synergy of people and place is the experiential field: body and space are no longer separate entities but exist in exchange and fusion (Mallgrave 2013). To explain how I arrived at a definition of the experiential field in a Maggie's centre, I refer to the one based on Merleau-Ponty's theory of the 'phenomenal field' or 'space of experience' investigated within the research "Dynamics of architectural experience in the perceptual field" developed by the scientist Sergei Gepshtein (ANFA) and the architect Tatiana Berger, presented virtually at the Amps "Experiential Design" conference, held in Florida in January 2020, where I too participated first-hand with my research on the Maggie's centre.

Gepshtein and Berger start from the architectural interpretation of the 'psychological field' of Gestalt psychology—which, as seen, had already influenced Merleau-Ponty—described by the Gestalt-trained art psychologist Rudolf Arnheim—already encountered in Chapter 2—in his book *The Dynamics of Architectural Form* (1977).

Arnheim points out that the spaces surrounding buildings cannot be considered empty. Instead, the spaces appear rated by visual forces generated by the architectural structures. He says further that visual forces should be understood as components of perceptual fields that surround buildings. He talks about these forces as dynamical processes that expand from their sources and propagate as if they had weight, as if they had quantifiable strength. Evidently, Arnhem uses the terms of force and field metaphorically.

(Gepshtein and Berger, 2020a, 15:05)

As Gepshtein clarifies, Arnheim does not use the terms 'force' and 'field' in a scientific way but only abstractly, since it is not clear how correlated entities can be measured and how the structure of the proposed experience can be validated. However:

Today the sciences have provided us with the tools to understand the human body, the behavior of the brain and how the built environment influences the user experience (...) scientific methods can help reveal the hidden structure of experiential fields and help us predict sequences of experiences.

(Gepshtein and Berger, 2020a, 12:55)

To illustrate it, Arnheim uses a drawing by Paolo Portoghesi—which, for the same purpose, Gepshtein reproduces in his presentation—a planimetric diagramme of a building in which thick curved lines represent solid walls and thin concentric circles represent the effects of these walls on the observer (Figure 6.3). Finding the drawing extremely powerful and wanting to use it myself to illustrate to the reader the effect of the phenomenal field on the observer, I decided to go to the source. So, on 1 February 2023, I went to Calcata (Rome) and visited Paolo Portoghesi—unfortunately passed away on 30.05.2023—who explained to me how he met Arnheim in Rome and gave him the drawing, as well as the origin of his own study which found application and point of arrival in his project for the church of the *Sacra Famiglia*, built in Fratte (Salerno) in 1974. If you want to experience a phenomenal field, I invite everyone to visit this building. From a spatial point of view, the interior is a sort of 'magnetic' field made of visible and palpable concentric wavy circles, which, in a continuous and repetitive motion, follow one another and expand to infinity. Seeming to arise from a beating heart in the centre that rhythms the breath according to the observer's movement, space accompanies our emotional reactions.

When you enter the church you understand the difference between emotions and feelings, between poetry and the reason that conceived it.

(Priori, 2022, p. 29)

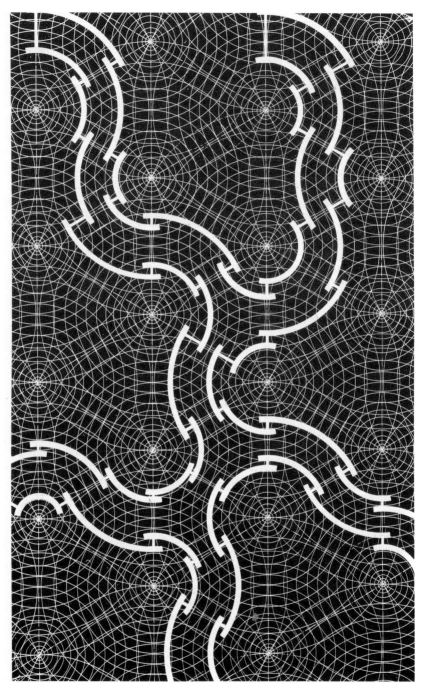

FIGURE 6.3 Planimetric diagramme of the Church of Fratte (1974) by Paolo Portoghesi, used by Rudolf Arnheim in his book (1977) to represent a hypothetical phenomenal field generated by the forces released by the curved walls (Courtesy of Paolo Portoghesi).

Since the 1960s, Paolo Portoghesi had developed a theory of design, "the space as a system of places", an attempt to give control over the form and, at the same time, to give the architecture a social consideration (*Portoghesi, 01.02.2023*).

> None of us is really alone, each of us exists as the others exist, which is also confirmed by science and by the famous mirror neurons which are a bit of proof of it. On this I wanted to build an architectural control system which, at the same time, would allow for the exploration of what architecture had not yet explored, namely the use of the curve to shape space.
>
> (*Portoghesi, 01.02.2023**)

For Portoghesi an essential architectural element for architecture such as the wall becomes part of relationships, acquiring its maximum spatial potential when it curves. "When the wall inflects, this strange fact occurs: the space compresses on one side and expands on the other which, for the architect, is an extraordinary resource" (*01.02.2023*). For architects, believing that the space between two buildings is not empty but forms a field of forces that spreads from the walls of each building—giving rise to a complex system of spatial overlapping—is as important as believing that it is the sun that revolves around the earth and not—pretending to ignore the Copernican theory—the other way around. In this, the wall takes on a crucial role thanks to its 'fixity'—honouring the sun with its shadows—in generating dynamism in space. In sensory perception, dynamics, as Arnheim had understood, is the deciding factor. And in order for this to be possible, an object needs to be adequately perceived by the observer, i.e. the field of forces propagated by its walls must be respected by the observer placing himself/herself at the right distance (Arnheim, 1977).

Based on this last insight and believing that the space of experience could be implemented in valid scientific terms, starting from previous psychophysical studies which had led to the formulation of some laws of perception, Gepshtein went further and managed, using a simple model, to confirm in detail "how our ability to see objects depends on distance between the observer and the object" (Kelly, 1979, Watson and Ahumada, 2016, quoted in Gepshtein and Berger, 2020, p. 89). Just as the physical walls of a building separate the inside from the outside, the boundaries of experience separate the parts of the space where an object is visible from the parts where it is not visible. According to Gepstein, the boundaries of experience in the illustrated model derive from the person's biological limits, and are spatial manifestations of the person's body. In short, the space thus described is what the phenomenologist calls an 'embodied space', opposed to the notion of empty space between buildings. As Berger explains:

> The space surrounding the body is not empty or neutral. It is a dynamic perceptual field, shared by the body and the built environment. (...) The experience is multisensory in its very essence, but it also involves perception beyond the five Aristotelian senses, building upon the sensations of orientation, gravity, balance, duration, and stability, of which many arise through movement.
>
> (Gepshtein and Berger, 2020b, pp. 90–91)

As for Merleau-Ponty experiencing space requires "a more active form of vision" which depends on maintaining bodily movement (2012 [1945], p. 249), for Gepshtein and Berger, experiential fields "by their very nature, encourage movement and invite exploration by the observer" (2020, 23:55). Due to movement, the experience of space is always sequential and "forms a spatial temporal structure" (2020, 23:25). The body, moving in space and continuously changing position, feels a new experience every time in a sequence of ever-changing positions. Perceived with the whole body, in turn, the space changes at all times depending on the position of the observer, allowing for a fusion, i.e. an 'embodied experience'.

While requiring scientific validation, Gepshtein's experiment has ultimately demonstrated how it is actually possible to translate psychophysical laws from laboratory conditions into conditions of human immersive experience moving in space and how scientific methods are able to "reveal the hidden structure of experiential fields" confirming the definition of "structured arena" intuited by Merleau-Ponty (1963 [1942]). After adding a "layer of concreteness" to the "layer of philosophical reflection" of the concept of "space of experience", together with Berger, Gepshtein concludes:

> We suggested how spatial thought in architecture could use elements of scientific exploration, which implies that we carefully separate intellectual and experiential species of space. This way, we began uncovering the hitherto hidden structure of space of experience, for which mobility is an essential condition.
>
> (Gepshtein and Berger, 2020b, pp. 93–94)

Fascinated by the idea that "the spaces appear rated by visual forces generated by the architectural structures" and of being able to "reveal the hidden structure of experiential fields"—which for an architect is a sort of grid—and finally by "how methods from science can help us predict sequences of experiences", following the description of the phenomenological field given by Gepshtein and Berger (2020), I returned to the interviews with Maggie's architects to make sure they were aware that in their project they had generated an experiential field.

Referring to his project for Maggie's West London (2008), Ivan Harbour (RSHP) had already explained to me how in a Maggie's centre the sequence of spaces divides or joins in a flexible way through sliding doors and movable walls "which can be left a little open".

> What I learnt from Laura and Marcia inspired the spatial experience; they wanted the ability to find protected space within a larger space, which in itself also—how can I describe this—gives an extended experience. In other words, the building, whatever one said, was not really a set of rooms, it's an evolving space and that was manifest in specific things Laura and Marcia said, such as 'we don't like doors that you close, we like to slide doors, because they can be left a little open'. I can say all of the spatial decisions that we took are based

upon the idea of continuity interspersed, a sort of evolving experience. You read that physically in obvious things such as 'the building as a grid'.

(*Harbour, 20.07.2018*)

Surprisingly similar to the description of the 'experiential field' made by Gepshtein and Berger, Harbour's account finds further correspondence in the description that the two speakers provided of Peter Zumthor's project for the Thermal Baths at Vals in Switzerland, brought as an example of 'sensory field'.

Adjacent locations offer the person different experiences and sensory motor affordances, thus creating a continuous field. (…) In this building we never see the entire structure or a dominant form at once, but we sense it gradually over time with our body through the texture, temperature and colour of the stone, the sound of water, the overall ambience. Here's what Zumthor wrote about the building: 'Moving around this space means making discoveries, you're walking, as if in the woods. The stone rooms were designed not to compete with the body, but to flatter the human form and give it space, room in which to be'.

(Gepshtein and Berger, 2020a, 23:50)

What Berger describes for Vals as "adjacent locations [that] offer the person different experiences and sensory motor affordances, thus creating a continuous field", we also find in a Maggie's centre. Harbour explains that when you look at Maggie's West London in plan, it could be an office building, it's just an open 'grid' and it's used quite 'dramatically' (Figures 6.4 and 6.5). "There is nothing romantic about it" in the way that it's being envisaged, but it is the spatial continuity together with that of the treatment which allows it to "stand as a neutral background to the activity".

In addition to the continuity of the spaces, what contributes to creating an experiential field is the continuity of the light which reinforces the perception of the continuous space.

I think, one of the most important aspects of the building is the 'clear through', because you understand of course that the space is continuous, even though what breaks the space up is the thing that actually defines the local moment. And the continuity of the way that the moments are defined in materially, you know they are basically, the sort of bookshelves that divide everything up, is also continuous.

(*Harbour, 20.07.2018*)

At Maggie's West London (2008), in this seamless and ever-changing space, if we look up, we can see a floating roof with lanterns framing the clouds visually mitigating the intrusive presence of the hospital (Figures 6.5 and 6.6). In Maggie's Aberdeen (2013), where, upon entering, "our eyes are attracted to the ceiling by colored skylights", the light spreads in the open and round space radiating vital energy (*Aabø, 02.11.2018*) becoming "material, spatial and visible"

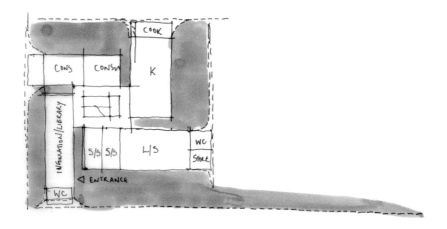

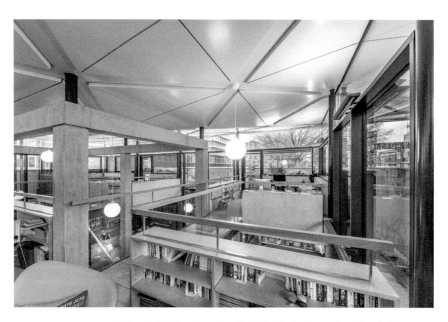

FIGURES 6.4 AND 6.5 Maggie's West London (2008). Early floor plan sketch (Courtesy of RSHP). At Maggie's the idea of an interspersed continuity, a kind of evolving experience, is physically readable in obvious things like "the building as a grid" (©Marco Castelli Nirmal).

at Maggie's Barts, because "light and space are inextricable from each other" and "the beauty of light is its energy" (*McVoy, 05.26.2018*).

After having activated the 'feeling of the place' and the factors that contribute to it—then all the sensors such as space, light and materials that generate a sensory space—since sensory experience involves perception beyond the five senses, Maggie's architects go further, making the sensory space an experiential field. In the difficult phase of designing an experiential field, which harmoniously accompanies

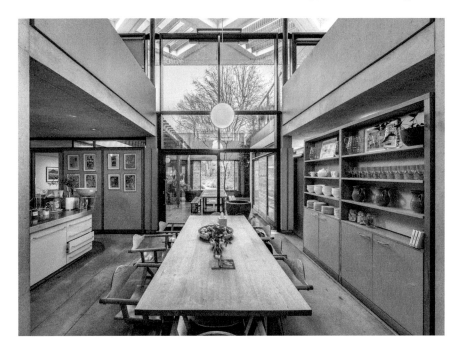

FIGURE 6.6   At Maggie's West London (2008), if we look up we can see a floating roof with lanterns framing the clouds visually mitigating the intrusive presence of the hospital (©Marco Castelli Nirmal).

the movement of the body making the person *feel included, at home and valued*, the architectural project of a Maggie's centre is fundamentally a human-centred design model, and Harbour explains it very well. But what is more difficult for a Maggie's architect to interpret is the 'non-said' of the Architectural Brief and, as Harbours says, the slightest misreading "between the lines" can make all the difference.

> Personally, I approach all of my work based upon what I see as the human experi-
> ence. For me that is the number one priority in architecture and it's really hard to
> put your finger on what makes that. That's the alchemy. But also, I'm not purport-
> ing 'to know how', it comes, I think, out of trying to understand what the problem
> is. So, there is a 'problem-solving' part, 'how you put that together and make a
> place that feels good', and it's that. It's the feel of the place and the contribu-
> tors to that feeling are everything from the way that—as we've talked about the
> senses—all the senses, so it's acoustics, it's light, and the materials, textures and
> colours. So, it's everything from end to end that deliver that. But what is really in-
> teresting is how there's a very fine balance between doing that really successfully
> and not achieving it, it's such a fine balance. The difference can be a small thing.
> (*Harbour, 20.07.2018*)

Reading in Harbour's 'small thing' the "essential component of the spatial experience" described by Gepshtein and Berger, in full harmony with their suggestion to

take further steps in investigating "how the architect could use explicit knowledge about boundaries of experience in the process of design", it would seem that Maggie's architects, in addition to being aware that there is an experiential field in their project, are oriented towards welcoming the help of "specific tools" to promote an interweaving of science and human-centred design thinking which, at Maggie's, has already given birth to the new discipline advocated by Gepshtein and Berger.

> All in all, it appears that the architectural profession needs to bring the full-blooded human being into its very core. (…) Sooner or later, the 'human sciences' will intertwine with every step of architectural and urban design. (…) As the profession moves from the abstract object-oriented design to humanistic experience driven design, here we have described an attempt to advance studies of experience towards specific tools that can be used in practice. (…) This is just one illustration of how space can be conceived in a framework that puts human experience in a centre. We suspect that pursuing this line of inquiry will amount to a new discipline that will be as different from pure scientific practice as it is, from traditional architectural practice.
>
> (Gepshtein and Berger, 2020a, 25:35)

What Originates the Experiential Field

At Maggie's, the space of experience is enabled by a variety of solutions that create movement, which we know is the key element that allows flexibility and that connects architecture to psychological flexibility. But where does the movement come from? And what exactly is it about the architecture that triggers it? Knowing that the projects of the Maggie's centres are the result of the application of the Architectural Brief, if we carefully examine the document, we discover that the request for 'movement' is already implicit in the first requirement. The continuous space, visible from the welcome area, invites us to walk (Appendix I).

> *Entrance:* clear, welcoming, not intimidating. Small coat-hanging / brolly space. A welcome / sitting / information / library area from which the layout of the rest of the building should be clear. There should be as much light as possible. There should be views of grass / trees / sky. You should be able to see where the kitchen area is, equally the sitting room and fireplace-area (hearth & home). Maggie suggested a fish tank.
>
> (Maggie's Brief, 2007, p. 2)

Once inside, depending on the mood of the individual and thanks to the seamless spatial sequence, people looking for social interaction will let themselves be attracted by the noise coming from the kitchen; if, on the other hand, they want a quieter environment, they will be called by a more secluded space such as the library or the garden. If we continue to analyse the entire Architectural Brief, we realise that movement is a constant reminder throughout the text (Figure 6.7).

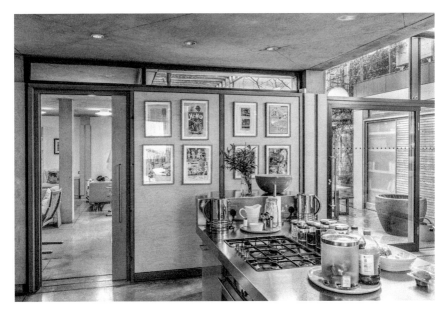

FIGURE 6.7   At Maggie's the sequence of spaces divides or joins in a flexible way through sliding doors and movable walls 'which can be left a little open' (Maggie's West London, 2008) (©Marco Castelli Nirmal).

> Kitchen should be relaxed and inviting enough for anybody to feel welcome (…) A large room for relaxation groups / lectures / meetings (…) you should be able to open and shut walls (perhaps between this and welcome area / kitchen area) to have flexi-space, (…) small rooms for counselling or therapy (…) have sliding doors that can be left open and be inviting when not in use. Furthermore, it is important to be able to look outside – and even get out (…) We want visitors to have an idea of what is going on in the whole building when they come in.
>
> (Maggie's Brief, 2007, pp. 2–5)

The sequence of spaces divides or joins flexibly through sliding doors and movable walls. The spatial experience is that of an evolving space, which encloses a space within a larger space, thus generating an extended experience. Going beyond the Architectural Brief, by way of curved glass cases, bending walls, and round spiral stairs, Maggie's architects are able to move people's bodies within a charged and changing space that surrounds the body. In the process of designing a Maggie's centre, "generators of architectural atmospheres", i.e. the combination of materials, light, colour and shape of the buildings (Martin, Nettleton and Buse, 2019) are certainly important to stimulate the senses, but not enough to explain the positive experience of Maggie's visitors. Since "the space of experience can only be understood by recognising that perceivers are freely moving individuals" (Gepshtein and Berger, 2020, 25:14), only by looking at the movement that Maggie's architects generate in the experiential field that pushes people's bodies, making them live an 'embodied experience', we begin to understand why and where the phenomeno-logical synergy that allows psychological flexibility in Maggie's visitors arises. To explain, however, what activates the movement that enables the experiential field, and therefore the true origin of the therapeutic power of the Maggie's centre, we must look to the architecture as a "desirable void" (Zucchi, 2020), i.e. to its 'clear through' (*Harbour, 20.07.2018*). As Le Corbusier had intuited in regard to his *promenade architecturale*, what generates movement, releasing to the observer a sequence of images that constitute "a set of instructions for reading the work, the 'internal circulatory system' of architecture" (Samuel, 2010, p. 6), is *transparency*.

From the Latin verb *trans-parere*, 'transparency' literally means to 'appear through'. With the assumption that we are all sighted, transparency is not only an inherent quality of a clear glass; in architecture, transparency is a way of organis-ing space that gives us a reading on multiple levels. Already in 1956, in their essay *Transparency: literal and phenomenal*, Colin Rowe and Robert Slutzky argued that transparency is not that of the Bauhaus glass (literal), but that which is ob-tained empirically from Le Corbusier's Villa Garche (phenomenal). In reporting the definition of this condition to be discovered in a work of art given by Gyorgy Kepes—educator and art theorist who had taught theory of light and colour at the New Bauhaus in Chicago founded in 1937 by László Moholy-Nagy—Rowe and Slutzky report that transparency is more than an optical feature.

> If one sees two or more figures overlapping one another, and each of them claims for itself the common overlapped part, then one is confronted with a con-tradiction of spatial dimensions. To resolve this contradiction, one must assume the presence of a new optical quality. The figures are endowed with transpar-ency; that is, they are able to interpenetrate without an optical destruction of each other. Transparency however implies more than an optical characteristic; it implies a broader spatial order. Transparency means simultaneous perception of different spatial locations. Space not only recedes but fluctuates in a continuous activity. The position of the transparent figures has equivocal meaning as one sees each figure now as the closer now as the further one.
>
> (Kepes, 1944, quoted in Rowe and Slutzky, 1963 [1956], p. 33)

Constantly perceiving "transparent overlapping planes" rather than mere physical transparency, the "transparent ceases to be that which is perfectly clear [literal] and becomes instead that which is clearly ambiguous [phenomenal]". According to Rowe and Slutzky, achieving phenomenal transparency is difficult, so difficult that critics have generally associated transparency in architecture solely with the transparency of materials. On the contrary, Kepes tells us that in architecture trans-parency must be sought in the random overlaps produced by "the reflections and accidents of light playing upon a translucent or polished surface". These stratifica-tions, these devices with which the space "becomes constructed, substantial and articulated", are the essence of that phenomenal transparency adopted by Maggie's architects, a "small thing" (*Harbour, 20.07.2018*) (Figures 6.8 and 6.9).

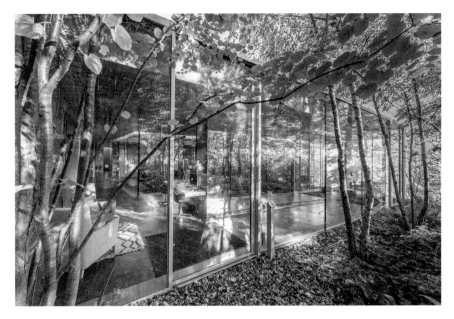

FIGURE 6.8   At Maggie's, stratifications of images are the essence of phenomenal transparency (Maggie's Glasgow, 2011) (©Marco Castelli Nirmal).

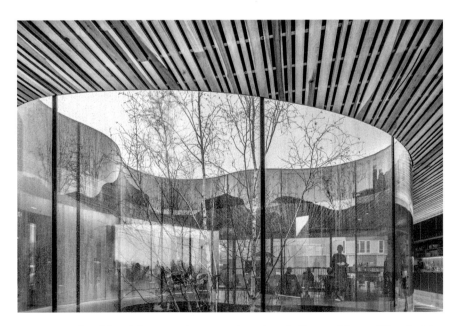

FIGURE 6.9   In a Maggie' centre, phenomenology is an indispensable condition for triggering psychological flexibility (Maggie's Oldham, 2017) (©Marco Castelli Nirmal).

Within a charged and ever-changing space where cuts of light or, vice versa, surfaces with diffused light allow long perspectives that convey a sense of control, *transparency* makes us understand that space is continuous (*Harbour, 20.07.2018*). The interchangeability of continuous space, i.e. "the idea of continuity interspersed", a vague continuity—where vague, from the Latin term *vagus* (=wandering, strolling), stimulates curiosity—is what drives movement in "a sort of evolving experience". Going beyond the senses, with "a more active form of vision" and renewing each act of focusing (Merleau-Ponty 2012 [1945], p. 249), the transparency of the experiential field, full of forces that move and make it so that "the observer fuses with the space" (Gepshtein and Berger, 2020b, p. 87) allowing for an 'embodied experience' and facilitating emotions ("I don't know how to explain it"), is the key to understanding the therapeutic power of the Maggie's centre.

In the therapeutic process, seen as a development from cancer to psychological flexibility, passing through the experiential field, Maggie's transparency, characterised by "the reflections and accidents of light playing upon a translucent or polished surface", is what involves the visitors who, as they move through the space, feel connected, even amused at being able to wave from one side to the other. This means that, in the therapeutic process, phenomenology is an indispensable condition for triggering psychological flexibility, as well as enabling a sense of identity, which encourages people to feel active, in control and normal, which is why at Maggie's the person with cancer says: "When I'm at Maggie's I don't feel like I'm in hospital, I don't feel like a patient" (*Focus-group Oldham*).

Movement and 'Embodied Experience'

At Maggie's, visitors are encouraged to go wherever they want to experience the place. Since they are not familiar with the building when they first arrive, newcomers unconsciously employ spatial resolution practices such as *wayfinding* (Lynch, 1960). As Sarah Williams Goldhagen tells us in her book *Welcome to Your World* (2017a), in our brain we have an "internal GPS" that allows us to orient ourselves in space and, thanks to Lynch's work, carried out by a group of cognitive neuroscientists—2014 Nobel Prize winners O'Keefe, Britt-Moser, Moser—today we know we have it. The three neuroscientists in fact discovered in rats moving freely in a room, first, the activation of certain nerve cells in the hippocampus that they called "place cells" (O'Keefe, 1976) and then, a cluster of another type of nerve cell in the entorhinal cortex, that they called "grid cells" (Hafting et al., 2005). The 'place' and the 'grid' cells form a circuit that constitutes a complete positioning system—an internal GPS—which demonstrates a cellular foundation for superior cognitive function (Williams Goldhagen, 2017a). This function is our ability to orient ourselves in space or to have knowledge of the place, where cognition—from the Latin verb *cognosco* (=con 'with' + gnōscō 'know') and from the Greek verb γιγνώσκω (=I know)—means to learn, know, or investigate.

During spatial navigation, thanks to the internal GPS—also found in humans through brain imaging techniques and studies on patients undergoing neurosurgery—our brain recognises landmarks such as paths, edges and junctions that we rely on to orient us in places we do not know; unconsciously we develop an internal 'cognitive map' to which images of the external environment correspond. With the discovery of 'place-recognition cells', it is now clear why patients with Alzheimer's disease—which initially affects the hippocampus and entorhinal cortex—become lost and unable to recognise their surroundings (Williams Goldhagen, 2017a). In elaborating their cognitive map, people implement the ability to imagine 'associatively' and, therefore, to associate previous events. For example, at Maggie's, by connecting the typical elements of a place, such as the kitchen, Maggie's visitors immediately recognises a warm and comfortable environment that makes them move around with ease.

With *wayfinding*, perception goes beyond the five senses and becomes an 'embodied experience'. In a blind person, this fact is even more striking because in addition to developing all the other senses—especially touch and hearing—the whole body becomes the main receptor. At the same conference in Florida organised by Amps (2020) mentioned above, the keynote lecture was given by Chris Downey, an architect from San Francisco who went blind in 2008 following a brain operation. In addition to giving hope to many disabled people of being able to continue carrying out their job despite serious physical limitations, his story (which I found online from other sources as the conference speech is not available) is testimony of how, when immersed in the built environment, the body perceives holistically and not with vision.

It was very unexpected. I lost my sight in surgery to remove a brain tumour. An essential part of dealing with my blindness was embracing the challenge. That's sort of that leap of faith you have to take as a designer, as an architect. You never know what the answer is, but you have to believe in the process. Within a month of losing my sight, I went back to the office to start figuring it out. With new technologies, I can take architectural drawings and print them in tactile form. When I'm reading a floor plan of the building, my mind is actively thinking about all the materials, the composition, the warmth the sun coming to the window, all sorts of things that are always there, available to my mind. But in reading drawings with my eyes, I was more passive. [Now] I'm always very careful to say that I went outside not without vision. My idea of vision is to see with more than just your eyes.

(Downey, 2013, 0:50)

As Chris explains, when you lose your sight you realise that the experience becomes much more multisensory than the sighted experience ever was. Furthermore, by knowing about the environment, one learns to pay close attention to what is on the ground and to the sounds bouncing off buildings around you "when you pass a building, because all of a sudden that reverb that used to be there opened up and you're hearing something else off in the distance". In his *wayfinding* experience, thanks to the reflection of the sound, Chris Downey is even able tell how high the ceiling of a room is. For him, the point is that it's not the loss of sight that prevents us from having a multisensory experience, rather it is the unawareness of our ability to organise our environment in a "completely different way". Inviting architects to reflect on it, this "completely different way" could find application in architecture helping anyone to have an 'embodied experience'.

> Once I really understand the space that I'm dealing with, it's almost as if my feet are at the tip of my fingers. And as I'm reading the drawing, I'm in the space. And I can imagine the space around me, the walls, the materials; like: can you imagine what it sounds like? And it starts to suggest ways of how to design in the space working with making difference in the acoustics, making difference out of a tactile palette of materials, not just a colour palette, the metallic materials and all the ways to work with, all these different things so that you really create a much more rich, multisensory environment that really recognise the difference between architecture and graphic design. That it's a place for your whole body and your whole being, a place to be, not just a place to look at.
>
> (Downey, 2012, 12:34)

The way of designing a multisensory space 'for your whole body' is the one I have been describing until now about the Maggie's centre. Trying to imagine what architects and neuroscientists might learn from the lesson of Chris Downey—who wonders, as patient, designer and user of his buildings, "if all the other architects out there are obsessed with 'what this thing looks like', where do I fit into that?" (Downey, 2012, 12:00), but who is also determined to commute "to work on my own, walking through town" (Downey, 2013, 3:40)—I might think that architects would understand that we should no longer design only for the pleasure of 'sight', but for all the senses, i.e. for the human body as a whole receptor. Neuroscientists, on the other hand, would deduce that, despite blindness, human beings still need movement, which is how the body responds to the built environment. And this is because experiencing architecture while moving is essential to generate besides perception, a sense of identity. To this aim, we should remember that, in addition to controlling spatial navigation and containing what we now know to be 'place recognition' neurons, the hippocampus is the area of the brain where we consolidate long-term autobiographical memories. As Sarah Williams Goldhagen (2017a) argues, this means that we cannot develop a long-term memory of an experience that doesn't contain something of where we were when we had that experience. This discovery alone "means nothing less than architecture and the built environment are central to the formation of our identities" (Williams Goldhagen, 2017b, para. 10).

Representing a paradigm shift in our understanding of the world, the studies above and, in general, the resources that neuroscience offers us, have the potential to help us design a built environment that allows users to live an 'embodied experience', the same one described by Chris Downey who is always on the move. Paradoxically, thinking of the blind, we would be able to design an environment that makes one feel 'included', 'valued' and 'at home', the same conditions that at Maggie's give rise to feelings and emotions. And this is because, as seen in Chapter 2, no emotion can arise if it is not linked to movement (Berthoz, 2000).

In the next section I will provide a quick overview of the biology of emotions and feelings—which are active perceptions generated by movement—helping the reader to recognise, as suggested by Berthoz (2000), the relationship between movement and emotion, indicative of an architecture that makes one feel good. In this regard, Mallgrave (2013) reminds us that biological pleasure is not a feeling, but the result of a system which, by responding to environmental stimuli, judges and codifies the subjective and emotional relevance of pleasure and pain, that is, "whether something is 'good' or 'bad' for me" (Mallgrave, 2013, p. 47). According to Damasio (1994), knowing the biological mechanisms underlying emotions and feelings helps us, first of all, to know ourselves and then the environment that surrounds us. In short, feeling one's emotional states, that is, being aware of one's emotions and one's self, facilitates one's flexibility in responding to the environment. This leads to a new paradigm offered by the Maggie's centre which, open to any interpretation and without claiming to heal anyone, suggests a model of flexibility to be applied, as we will see in the next chapter, to other healthcare and non-healthcare facilities and to architecture in general.

A Biology of Emotions and Feelings

Emotion tints all human experience.

(Tuan, 1977, p. 8)

As Marco Maiocchi of NAAD says, there is nothing romantic about emotions. "Emotion is the way in which Nature, the evolution of the species, has defined the ability to compete with other species, with greater chances of survival" (Maiocchi, 2017, 1:01). The first scientific research on emotions was that of Charles Darwin published in his book *The Expression of the Emotions in Man and Animals* (1872) showing the similarities of the expressions of the emotions in humans and animals. On this study, in 1960s, Paul Ekman developed his theory of *basic emotions*, according to which there is a limited number of emotions in the brain (fear, anger, disgust, surprise, sadness and happiness) whose corresponding facial expressions are indifferently common to cultures and ethnicities (Ekman, Sorenson, and Friesen, 1969). While, as Damasio (2004) tells us, there are also other types of emotions—such as *background emotions* and *social emotions*—the commonalities between ethnic groups of *basic emotions* explain why neurobiological research has mainly focused on them, yet associating them to less developed regions of the brain, neglecting the connection with the reasoning (Damasio, 1994).

As for feelings—which must be distinguished from emotions—again according to Damasio (2004), for a long time, neuroscience even excluded them from the academic curriculum: everything was permissible to study except feelings, because they were considered elusive and therefore destined to remain mysterious. This reticence in addressing the subject was not only due to opponents who feared that neuroscience could discover "anything mental", but to the same neuroscientists who proclaimed "allegedly insurmountable limitations", without admitting that, instead, knowing the biology of feelings and emotions—which are an expression of human wellbeing or malaise—means better understanding "the state of life within the entire organism", as well as "the mind-body problem, a problem central to the understanding of who we are". In more practical terms, understanding the biology of feelings and emotions helps us discover "some major causes of human suffering" (Damasio, 2004, pp. 4–7).

While we tend to think that the concept of emotion contains that of feeling and that "the hidden is the source of the expressed" favouring the idea that feelings manifest themselves before emotions, for Damasio this view is wrong. "It turns out that it is feelings are mostly shadows of the external modality of emotions" (2004, p. 30); and this is because, in developing life's governing apparatus— the homeostasis machine—human evolution first allowed for emotions—that is, simple reactions to aid survival—just like crying and sobbing in a new-born that are ready for use at birth. In an attempt to explain the complicated chain of events that begins with emotion and ends with feeling, Damasio (2004) tells us that emotion takes place in the "theatre 'of the body' while feelings in that of the mind".

> Emotions are actions or movements, many of them public, visible to others as they occur in the face, in the voice, in specific behaviours. (…) Feelings, on the other hand, are always hidden, like all mental images necessarily are, unseen to anyone other than their rightful owner, the most private property of the organism in whose brain they occur.
>
> (Damasio, 2004, p. 28)

Damasio (2004) describes an emotion as a complex of biochemical and neural responses; these responses are automatic, always as a result of evolution, giving the brain that perceives a stimulus, a specific repertoire of actions. The immediate result of these responses is a temporary change in the body proper and in the state of the brain structures that map the body and support thinking. The final result of these responses is to place the organism in conditions of survival and wellbeing. "What we identify as wellbeing is, in fact, an effort of homeostasis to provide a better than neutral state of life" (2004, p. 35). All these phenomena refer to the adaptation of the body state and ultimately lead to changes in the brain mapping of body states, on which feelings are based (Damasio, 2004).

Among brain structures, the *cerebral cortex* is the one to which neuroscience has devoted itself most. As Damasio (1994) describes it, it's a multi-layered blanket about 3 mm thick and all grey matter below it (nuclei, large and small, and the cerebellar cortex) is known as *subcortical*. Nervous (or neural) tissue is made of nerve cells (*neurons*), which are the cells essential for brain activity. In our brain we have billions of neurons, organised in local circuits, which form cortical *regions* (if arranged in layers) or *nuclei* (if arranged in non-layered ensembles). A division of the cortical and subcortical central nervous system known as the *limbic system* is the one that deals with emotions (Damasio, 1994).

As mentioned above, the emergence of an emotion depends on a complicated chain of events. The chain begins with a stimulus, a certain object or situation/ image actually present or recalled from memory, which comes to mind. In neural terms, stimulus-related images must be represented in one or more sensory processing systems of the brain, such as visual or auditory regions. In simple terms, in the case of a memory, even if we think of it as a single image, it is actually the sum of many images (images are not only visual, they are also auditory, olfactory and so on) that come to mind from different regions: sound comes from the auditory region, sight from the visual one, etc. (Damasio, 1994). The olfactory regions are particularly active especially when stimulated by memory, which plays an important role in evoking emotions when we smell (Bear, Connors and Paradiso, 2016). As Maggie's users say, implying that they feel at home, "Maggie's doesn't smell like a hospital, it doesn't smell like an anaesthetic. She smells good, she smells like a home-cooked meal" (*Volunteer_no.6 Barts*). It is no coincidence that the kitchen table brings to users' minds memories capable of a mix of emotions. "So many conversations, so many laughs and some tears as well" (*Move-along_no.2 Dundee*).

An emotion involves a framework of three reactions to an event: physiological, behavioural, and cognitive. For example, if an event surprises us, there may be a change in facial expression or tone of voice, an increase in heart rate or breathing which leads us to change our body posture (with symptoms of freezing, flushing, sweating), and to think positively or negatively for a certain period of time. If emotions are not too strong or we are balanced people, the emotional region of the brain that comes into play before the thinking one is then inhibited by reason and everything falls back quickly. Sometimes, however, the brain's emotional reactions are so strong they dominate our behaviour and we are unable to think rationally (Lazarus and Folkman, 1984). Recalling the example of the stressful experience lived in the doctor's office recounted in Chapter 5 can help to understand what Maggie's visitors experience when they go to the hospital. In listening to their story, as well as understanding from their voice that the mere memory of an event aroused the same stressful emotions in them, I became aware of this inability to think clearly.

> When you're, when you're over the hospital, the control is kind (…), a lot of times you can't, you don't have much control. But when you come in here, you can control the level of whatever you want. If you want to let emotions go, you can do that, if you want. So, it's like 'I can', 'it's my choice', I can do that, and I can feel safe to do that, here. When you're over there, sometimes you have to listen so carefully to what's going on. So, you grasp or regulate.
>
> (*Follow-up Dundee*)

To create an emotional state, signals related to a stimulus are activated in a number of 'triggering-sites' which, through 'neural connections' (humans have several trillion of them), transmit their activity to the 'executive-sites' located in other parts of the brain. Among many 'emotion-triggering sites', the *amygdala* (part of the limbic system)—which, in our case, is important to know because it is a crucial interface between visual and auditory stimuli and the activation of emotions such as 'fear' and 'anger'—can detect stimuli very quickly and unconsciously. This explains why even in a person with a blind field of vision, emotionally competent stimuli, such as angry or happy faces, are able to "break-through" the barrier of blindness and, bypassing the normal process, actually being detected, causing emotions to arise. Among the 'emotion-execution sites', the *hypothalamus* controls those physiological changes that occur automatically without us being able to control them (sweating, rapid breathing, accelerated heartbeat) and, through the pituitary gland, releases chemical molecules into the bloodstream, altering the function of the body and of the nervous system itself (Damasio, 2004). In stressful situations, the hormone released is *cortisol*, which prepares us for action, i.e. 'fight or flight'; in a calm environment or when we receive good news that gratifies us, the hormones involved are *serotonin*, also called the 'happiness hormone', and *dopamine*, a neurotransmitter that controls the reward and pleasure centres of the brain (Skov, 2010, cited in Mallgrave, 2013, p. 48).

According to Damasio (2004), two things happen during the emotional process: (1) the flow of mental contents triggers emotional responses and (2) emotions manifest themselves. The final result of these responses—which constitute the emotions that then flow into feelings—as aforementioned, is to put the organism in conditions of wellbeing. To understand what exactly the feeling of *wellbeing* consists of— "what did that 'feeling well' consist of?"—Damasio (2004) invites us to imagine a condition of total physical wellbeing (i.e. lying on a beach, warmed by the sun, with perfect sea, temperature, and blue-sky all around). In this imaginary story, the place of the phenomenon was the body; however, "the feeling of wellbeing and absence of pain" was so widespread that "it was difficult to describe precisely where that was happening in the body" (Damasio, 2004, p. 84). Reminding us of what Maggie's visitors say when they first arrive at the centre— "I cannot explain it", that is, they don't know how to describe their feelings and where they come from—from what Damasio (2004) says, we understand that feelings arise not only from emotional labour, but also from the primary place of feeling, i.e. the body. As Damasio (2004) concludes in his story, a situation of physical wellbeing, derived from a perfect environmental condition all around, led to mental consequences, that is, the mind was fed with good thoughts which created further more positive thoughts in which the images were clear and flowed without haste. In short, "what you usually regard as 'body' and as 'mind' blended in harmony" (2004, p. 84), which is, ultimately, the feeling of *wellbeing*.

To confirm this idea, the neurobiologist 'Bud' Craig (2015, cited in Damasio, 2004) has made an important discovery. Of all the areas that influence feelings present at multiple levels of the central nervous system, the most important area of the brain is the hidden *insula*. Having understood that this region—which both theoretical and imaging studies relate to feelings—is the same region where the signals representing the content of feelings arrive—such as pain and body temperature, redness, itching, tickling, chills, etc.—'Bud' Craig (2015) discovered that we have an 'interceptive sense', a sense of the body. Deducing that 'somatosensory' (=of the body) brain regions are a critical substrate for feelings, 'Bud' Craig has demonstrated that whatever we 'feel' must be based on the activity pattern of the brain region that perceives the body.

According to Damasio (2004), feelings are perceptions and, in a way, comparable to other perceptions such as visual perception, where part of the phenomenon resides in an object and part in the internal construction of the brain. But while during the perception, for example, of a painting, the phenomenon can modify the emotion inside the observer but not the painting outside, in the case of perception as a feeling, since the object is inside the body (as parts and states of the living organism in which feelings arise), a feeling can also change the body proper. In other words, "feelings are not passive like perceptions", on the contrary, as a feeling arises, for a moment—seconds or minutes—the body is dynamically involved, almost certainly in repeatedly, determining a dynamic variation of perception. "We perceive a series of transitions. We sense an interplay, a give and take" (Damasio, 2004, p. 92).

Knowing that in a Maggie's centre visitors go through multiple moments of transition and that the immediate object of perception is the open space—which is not static but dynamic and which the observer is able to modify with its own movement—Damasio's statement leads us to say that the perception of Maggie's visitor, active and in movement, is indeed a 'feeling'. This fact, which confirms the existence of a physiology of relationships between movement and emotion (Berthoz, 2000), demonstrates that, in generating movement, the architecture of the Maggie's centre also generates emotions and feelings. And as an integral part of perception, "facial expression is a powerful indicator of emotion" (Berthoz, 2000, p. 188). As we will see in the last chapter, it is on the basis of emotions and feelings that in the future we will judge the built environment, according to a 'new way of perceiving architecture'.

References

Arnheim, R. (1977) *The Dynamics of Architectural Form*. Berkeley, Los Angeles, and London: University of California Press.

Bear, M. F., Connors, B. W. and Paradiso, M. A. (2016) *Neuroscienze. Esplorando il cervello*. Milan: Edra.

Berthoz, A. (2000) *The Brain's Sense of Movement*. Boston, MA: Harvard University Press

Boella, L. (2021) 'L'empatia, risorsa in un mondo in crisi'. https://www.youtube.com/watch?v=NpZPVIbxTNM&ab_channel=AssoCounseling

'Bud' Craig, A. D. (2015) *How Do You Feel? An Interoceptive Moment with Your Neurobiological Self*. Princeton, NJ: Princeton University Press.

Covey, S. R. (1989) *The 7 Habits of Highly Effective People: Restoring the Character Ethic*. New York: Simon & Schuster

Damasio, A. (1994) *Descartes' Error: Emotion, Reason, and the Human Brain*. London: Vintage

Damasio, A. (2004) *Looking for Spinoza. Joy, Sorrow and the Feeling Brain*. London: Vintage

Darwin, C. (1965 [1872]) *The Expression of the Emotions in Man and Animals*. Chicago, IL: Chicago University Press.

D'Avenia, A. (2018) '15. Piccola Filosofia per matti', *Corriere della Sera*, 7 May. https://www.corriere.it/alessandro-davenia-letti-da-rifare/18_maggio_06/15-piccola-filosofia-matti-alessandro-d-avenia-letti-da-rifare-f0c88e92-5130-11e8-b393-1dfa8344f8a7.shtml

De Botton, A. (2023) A Therapeutic Journey: Lessons from the School of Life. London: Penguin Books Ltd

Downey, C. (2012) 'Chris Downey—New Vision in Architecture'. https://www.youtube.com/watch?v=yiizM232Zak&ab_channel=TEDxTalks

Downey, C. (2013) 'An Architect's Story: Chris Downey'. https://www.youtube.com/watch?v=zrtfXDk0L8A&ab_channel=AIANational

Ekman, P., Sorenson, E. R. and Friesen, W. V. (1969) 'Pan-cultural Elements in Facial Displays of Emotion', *Science*, 164(3875), pp. 86–88

Gepshtein, S. and Berger, T. (2020a) *Dynamics of Architectural Experience in the Perceptual Field*, 16 January. https://www.youtube.com/watch?v=HI7s8OhZpT4&ab_channel=AMPS

Gepshtein, S. and Berger, T. (2020b) 'Dynamics of Architectural Experience in the Perceptual Field', in McLane, Y. and Pable, J. (eds.) *AMPS Proceedings Series 18.1. Experiential Design–Rethinking Relations between People, Objects and Environments*. Florida State University, FL, 16–17 January, pp. 83–94.

Hafting, T., Fyhn, M., Molden, S., Moser, M.B. and Moser, E.I. (2005) 'Microstructure of a Spatial Map in the Entorhinal Cortex', *Nature*, 436(7052), pp. 801–806

Hale, J. (2017) *Merleau-Ponty for Architects*. London and New York: Routledge

Hall, E. T. (1966) *The Hidden Dimension*. Garden City, NY: Doubleday

Held, K. (2003) 'Husserl's Phenomenological Method', in Rodemeyer, L. (ed. and transl.) *The New Husserl: A Critical Reader*. Bloomington: Indiana University Press, pp. 3–31.

Hensel, M. (2010) 'Performance-Oriented Architecture', *FORMakademisk,* 3(1), pp. 36–56

Koffka, K. (1935) *Principles of Gestalt Psychology*. London: Lund Humphries

Lazarus, R. S. and Folkman, S. (1984) *Stress, Appraisal, and Coping*. New York: Springer Publishing Company.

Lynch, K. (1960) *The Image of the City*. Cambridge, MA: MIT Press

Maiocchi, M. (2017) *Sound, Emotion and Architecture*, 13 December. https://www.youtube.com/watch?v=GJ0z9kLSF9I&t=68s&ab_channel=NAADMasterIuav%27Neuroscience AppliedtoArchitecturalDesign%27

Mallgrave, H. F. (2013) *Architecture and Embodiment. The Implications of the New Sciences and Humanities for Design*. London and New York: Routledge.

Martin, D., Nettleton, S. and Buse, C. (2019) 'Affecting Care: Maggie's Centres and the Orchestration of Architectural Atmospheres', *Social Science & Medicine*, 240, pp. 1–8

Merleau-Ponty, M. (1963 [1942]) *The Structure of Behaviour*. Translated by A. L. Fisher. Boston, MA: Beacon

Merleau-Ponty, M. (2012 [1945]) *Phenomenology of Perception*. Translated by D. A. Landes. Abington and New York: Routledge

O'Keefe, J. (1976) 'Place Units in the Hippocampus of the Freely Moving Rat', *Experimental Neurology*, 51(1), 78–109

Priori, G. (2022) 'Quando l'architettura diventa Poesia', in Bozzaotra, C. and Ciniglio, A. (eds) *Premio Campania Architettura, 2022. La Chiesa della Sacra Famiglia, Fratte, Salerno.* Napoli: Giannini Editore, pp. 28–30

Rowe, C. and Slutzky, R. (1963 [1956]) 'Transparency, Literal and Phenomenal'*, Perspecta,* 8, pp. 45–54

Samuel, F. (2010) *Le Corbusier and the Architectural Promenade.* Basel: Birkhäuser

Williams Goldhagen, S. (2017a) *Welcome to Your World: How the Built Environment Shapes Our Lives.* New York: Harper Collins

Williams Goldhagen, S. (2017b) 'How the Brain Works and What It Means for Architecture'. Interview with Sarah Williams Goldhagen. Interviewed by M. C. Pedersen for Common Edge, 20 July. https://commonedge.org/sarah-williams-goldhagen-on-how-the-brain-works-and-what-it-means-for-architecture/

7

MAGGIE'S AS A PARADIGM AND THE FUTURE OF THE ARCHITECTURE OF CARE

Maggie's as Emerging Paradigm

As mentioned in the introduction, today, the rate of cancer diagnoses in Britain has increased significantly; at the same time, science has made great advances that allow for a longer course of the disease and a higher survival rate.

> With new diagnoses rising 3% each year, there is a growing need for Maggie's centres and the evidence-based support they offer people during diagnosis, treatment and survival.
>
> (Maggie's Evidence, 2015, p. 1)

As many other diseases are now becoming chronic, and people are surviving through their illness, the NHS and other key stakeholders have realised that the new generations of hospitals and supportive facilities will need more facilities of various types to accommodate chronic or semi-chronic patients. Well aware of this, Charles Jencks would have wanted all chronic diseases (dementia, diabetes, heart disease, obesity, stroke and multiple sclerosis) to have a structure be just like the Maggie's centre, close to but independent from the hospital.

> My hope is that the hospital evolves in a direction that incorporates these kinds of centres but doesn't swallow them up: they should be administratively and culturally separate. We hope to have a Maggie's centre in every single large cancer hospital, developing one by one. We are complementary to them, yin and yang.
>
> (Jencks, 2015, para. 23)

In the private practice of architecture, Maggie's model has already had influence. As mentioned in Chapter 4, by interviewing Maggie's architects, I found out that

DOI: 10.4324/9781003244516-7

the experience of designing a Maggie's centre has had a big impact on other projects going on in their offices—for both medical and non-medical facilities—to which they have applied the human-centred design approach acquired or reinforced through such an experience. In addition to influencing projects of other clients, this attitude has also influenced the clients themselves, builders, project managers, contractors, consultants who have indirectly learned it and who, in turn, have passed this mindset on to others, in a domino effect.

> I suppose that the fairly simple theory is that Maggie's are just all these little things that tiny things that have had different ripples. It's not changing the whole thing, but it's rippling through, and the design is really important in terms of how it is done. At the same time, it has gone on to influence other projects that we're working on, our projects. So, our projects through the office have been helped, hugely. It has got two benefits. It has influenced the clients and the clients then started to say: 'let's improve things'. This is a remarkable model of influence. And all Maggie did was to say 'we'll build this tiny little thing, we'll plant this tiny seed'. And that little seed, which has already influenced architects and clients, will grow and change the world.
>
> (*Page, 01.10.2018*)

As an emerging paradigm, in private sphere, Maggie's model of influence works on expanding the concept of the 'Construction of Health' from the 'body' to the 'mind'. However, in the practice of architecture in public health, it has not yet been successful enough. In an attempt to promote the Maggie's centre as an emerging paradigm and to illustrate how a paradigm shift might occur, the following sections provide the reader with the definition of 'paradigm' and the comparison between the current model of architecture of care, the hospital, with the one offered by Maggie's. In thinking about where to extend it, beyond other chronic disease healthcare facilities, Maggie's seed could take root in other non-healthcare facilities such as homes for the elderly or community centres that support special needs. Extended to these structures, integrated into a *continuum* of an extended healthcare environment, in a logic of future 'Construction of Health', Maggie's model could make a leap of scale and be applied to a Maggie's Hospital, a human-centred facility like the hospitals of the past were.

A Paradigm Shift in the Architecture of Care

The most frequently cited definition of 'paradigm' was provided by Thomas Kuhn in *The Structure of Scientific Revolutions* (1962), in which he describes it as the "universally recognised scientific achievements that, for a time, provide model problems and solutions for a community of practitioners, i.e. what is to be observed and scrutinised" (Kuhn 1962, p. 10); in short, a scheme or model for understanding and explaining aspects of reality (Rosenberg, 1986). Paradigms are dynamic states rather than final responses, and as research continues, anomalies appear that ultimately lead to new understandings of reality and new paradigms (Kuhn, 1962). Kuhn argued that having a paradigm is a sign of maturity in the development of a discipline. It provides an organisational principle that allows the discipline to solve problems that, before then, would have been unsolvable without it (Rosenberg, 1986).

When, after a long process, a particular discipline transits from one paradigm to another, in Kuhn's terminology this passage is called 'scientific revolution' or 'paradigm shift'. The reason why Kuhn came up with this concept—and named it 'revolution'—was that he realised that, for a long time, science had looked at some specific phenomena in a certain way, but that, suddenly, that system of representation turned out to be false. Kuhn argued that scientific progress is not an evolution, but rather a series of peaceful interludes interrupted by violent intellectual revolutions, and that in these revolutions one conceptual worldview is replaced by another (Kuhn, 1962).

Establishing a paradigm requires a system in which a body of work is accepted by a community on the basis of something already present, which has already been put into practice in all the different phases of the process and which accepts changes. So, a paradigm can only be applied to a continuously evolving system (Kuhn, 1962). Today, Maggie's constant growth in a substantial number of centres constitutes an existing *corpus*, a field of action shared by a community, making Maggie's model an establishing paradigm that brings fundamental content to the continually evolving hospital ground. In particular, considering that in public health, the standardised method of commissioning the hospital project, commonly called 'Design by Committee'—deeply rooted and difficult to modify in the future—constitutes the most critical point of the hospital paradigm, Maggie's concise and dynamic way of commissioning architects through the Architectural Brief could constitute a significant reference for a change of perspective, urgent and relevant at this time. In my interview with Laura Lee and Marcia Blakenham, Marcia told me she was surprised when an architect once said to them:

> You know, people need help with their brief, because for example, these hospitals say they want to feel like a Maggie's centre, but they don't know what it really means. The architect, to make a good project, needs a good Brief, he needs hospitals to ask them to do the right things.
>
> (*Blakenham, 18.05.2019*)

Made up of too many members, the NHS 'Design by Committee' has no unifying plan or vision, and until hospitals filter the relationship between client and architect by electing a committee of a few members, projects will continue to be fragmented and repetitive.

> The project commissioned by a committee composed of many members, through a Brief that constantly presents the fractional nature of what each member of the committee requires, means for the architect that, to be able to succeed in his intent, he must respond to many, too many different requests. Whereas, by keeping the

management in the hands of a maximum of two or three people, using a clear and content Brief like ours, architects cannot 'distract themselves' from trying to respond to what is necessary, in an attempt to please everyone. You should keep them away from politics, you should keep them away from what the sponsor wants.

(Lee, 18.05.2019)

Furthermore, the architects called to design hospitals are always the same, because they are considered 'specialists'. Having a very narrow worldview, specialists dislike new ideas and are not inclined to modify it (*de Rijke, 17.12.2018*) and, therefore, they always repeat the same project. And unfortunately, from my conversations with Maggie's staff it emerged that, although other healthcare facilities such as Macmillan are slightly better equipped than the hospital, they are still clinical, noisy and also very limited in space, thus reducing the possibility of helping people from an emotional point of view.

I have worked in the NHS for 30 years as an oncology nurse with various positions, and for the last 17 years of my career I have worked as a Macmillan clinical nurse specialist. But in the last four years it's just got exceptionally busy with a lot of stress. And this was probably one of the reasons why I decided to retire. So, it's quite a different environment to work in than Maggie's. There is always a lot of noise and hustle and bustle. There is never enough space to sit and talk to people, in privacy. Sometimes you have to sit in the waiting room and it's just not appropriate. And there is a lot of space used for meetings in the consultation rooms and taken away that privacy you could use to talk to patients. You can still help, but it is very difficult to do so when you are in a busy clinical environment with grey walls and hard chairs, and a lot of noise surrounding you.

(CCS_no.3 Dundee)

Based on Alex de Rijke's personal experience, the hospital paradigm is still recognised for its well-known components: a mechanistic and specialist vision, protocol – orientation, elaborate feel and absence of design. As mentioned in Chapter 2, this condition originated from the change in the human relationship with the hospital which occurred at the end of the eighteenth century, as denounced by Foucault in his *The Birth of the Clinic* (1973 [1963]) and, after that, remaining the fundamental flaw of the hospital, the patient was always considered passive, and in inferior conditions. Today, despite there being a lot of talk about a return to the human dimension in the healthcare sector, hospital architecture continues to be considered a place for the 'machine' and not for the 'person' and this fact will not change as long as there are great economic interests on the part of the pharmaceutical sector and medical machinery industries and will not invest in design.

Not many hospitals you enter talk about design; they talk about being a machine and a process; yes, it's procedural. The message you understand is organisational, procedural, medical, surgical, chemical; you don't understand it as a three-dimensional expression of care and that's what Maggie's does. They say: 'design matters', don't they? That's what Maggie's does, as well as human contact and human care matters. Those are two areas that hospitals struggle with, you know they have care, but it's disguised as a process. The nurses really care and lots of people in hospitals really care a lot, but it's sometimes difficult to see it, because it's hidden by a process and institutionalised problems wearing uniforms, so you can't see the care of them, because it's disguised, it's disguised as a machine.

(*de Rijke, 17.12.2018*)

The obvious element that most contrasts and distinguishes the Maggie's centre from a hospital is, in fact, the design. When asked "why are hospitals so often horrible", during the Phil Gusack Talk at the 'Architects for Health' AGM at RIBA 2018, Henry Marsh responded that "hospitals are biological hazard areas; they are full of windowless spaces or high windows; multi bed bays are grotesque" adding that "it is extraordinary how much difference can be made by windows with views and natural light" (Marsh, 2018, para. 14, 22). Author of two best-sellers, *Do not harm. Stories of Life, Death, and Brain Surgery* (2014) and *Admissions: A Life in Brain Surgery* (2017) and as a staunch supporter of the NHS, throughout his long career as a neurosurgeon, Henry Marsh had a big say in trying to influence the quality of the hospital environment so as to impact the health of patients and staff. He believes there are several factors that cause patients to feel unwell in NHS hospitals, where they "rarely get peace, rest or quiet and never a good night's sleep" (Marsh, 2018, para. 5). On the one hand, people have a "terrible hunger" for healthcare and "an ideological faith in technology" so, like the ancients who built pyramids or large cathedrals as an expression of their "fear of death", today, for the same reason, we build hospitals that "are becoming so complex they are no longer humane" (Marsh, 2018, para. 18). On the other hand, despite not having a high opinion of healthcare architects, clients do have their own responsibilities. Indeed, Marsh's seven-year struggle to turn a ward balcony into a garden and deal "with a not very complimentary view of Arts Officers or Arts Committees" to put artwork on waiting room walls, proves that the road towards an 'Architecture of Care' in hospitals is still uphill.

To get out of this situation, a hypothesis launched at the "European Healthcare Design Congress, Salus 2021" would be to stop investing so much in hospitals and, rather, transform the hospital into a 'repair shop'. By considering it as the centre of an integrated network, by "domesticating" the services offered, the hospital would assist more and more people in their homes or communities, shifting the unequal doctor-patient relationship in favour of the patient. This means that, before an integrated healthcare model, we would need a cultural change—not easy to activate—even it would first be necessary to explain the concept of "integrated network", which is very widespread but unclear in its meaning. As understood by Gray (2021), a hospital network is not composed of 'hubs' and 'spokes'—like airline networks—but of centreless 'nodes', of which the 'hospital' is obviously a very important one, but the 'Maggie's centre' is a node of "pulsating knowledge and right philosophy" that must be connected to all community hospitals.

Within an integrated network system, a *continuum* of an extended healthcare environment, which must also integrate non-healthcare facilities, it is the task of the 'Constructor of Health'—the hospital—to collaborate with the other structures to become part of them rather than prevail over them. In this, if the hospital were willing to accept the criticism and do something about it, not only could the Maggie's centre concept be used as a model to other individual organisations, but the different Maggie's centres, in their own independent contexts, could trigger networks of local healthcare facilities, offering them multiple paradigms (*de Rijke, 17.12.2018*). Only when all healthcare facilities adopt a holistic model of support but, above all, an exemplary model of life in which people, staff and patients, look in the same direction thanks to a unifying and edifying architecture, will we be able to change people's worldview and activate the paradigm shift in the Architecture of Care.

> Yes, I'm positive about it, because a hospital is a machine typically isn't it; it's a machine that's supposed to fix problems. But everyone knows it creates other problems at the same time as not always fixing the problem itself. So, everyone knows that hospital is not the place to get well, it's time to change that.
>
> (*de Rijke, 17.12.2018*)

Having learnt what characterises the hospital paradigm during my interviews with architects and staff, when I went back to the data I had collected I was able to derive the themes that characterise the Architecture of Care at Maggie's and compare them with those of the old hospital paradigm. The comparison between the current paradigm of the hospital and that offered by Maggie's constitutes a potential shift in the worldview of Architecture of Care, as well as a new contribution to the 'Construction of Health' (Table 7.1).

TABLE 7.1 Architecture of Care. A Paradigm Shift in the 'Construction of Health'

Old Paradigm of the Hospital	*New Paradigm of Maggie's*
Mechanistic view	Mind-as-important-as-the-body view
Standardised design of sanitary architecture	Design devoid of signs of sanitary architecture
Large buildings with waste of space	Small buildings where space is well utilised
Non-sensory design (static)	Multi-sensory design (dynamic)
Mono-functionality / Hospital Art	Hybrid (Architecture, Art, Spiritual, Healing)
Landscape as decoration	Landscape for therapeutic effects
No nature-therapeutic connection through materiality	Nature-therapeutic connection through materiality
Procedural (Consent form)	Non-procedural (no registration form)
Doctor-patient hierarchy (passive patient)	'Empower the Patient' motto (active patient)
Segregated life model (staff and patients separated)	Integrated life model (staff and visitors together)

The transitions from one paradigm to the next are not like the swinging back and forth of a pendulum, but rather they embody the old paradigm and overcome it with a new dimension, a new way of 'seeing' old knowledge (Ferguson, 1980). For a discipline such as architecture which aims to design the built environment for the human being by acting by stratification and incorporation, this concept of a 'new way of seeing' by integrating old knowledge is central to Maggie's 'Co-Clients-Architect-Users' Triad, whose roots lie in the Greek healing temples and in the Benedictine Rule.

Maggie's Triad: A Paradigm for a New 'Commissioning of Architecture'

Of the 30 Maggie's centres that are currently active, all are functioning well on average and, as Charles Jencks argues, they are architecturally "superb". As discussed in Chapter 4, looking at the end of the chain, the verification of this fact comes from the level of user satisfaction, which at Maggie's is generally very high. To monitor it, Maggie's promotes the POE (Post Occupancy Evaluation), a survey of the building carried out by a researcher with the aim of evaluating the architect's work (RIBA, 2016). If done correctly, this research, in addition to technical-environmental, social, economic and sustainable data, releases useful information about the user experience. The POE, in fact, should also address more complex issues such as the sense of identity, ownership and belonging, just like the one done for Maggie's Nottingham (RIBA et al., 2017). In reality, the POE is much more frequently of a technical-practical nature. As highlighted in that of Maggie's Dundee, for example, in addition to the lack of storage, there are some technical problems of thermal and acoustic comfort linked to the design choice of having large glass surfaces and open spaces, problems common to all the centres as they derive from the requests of the Architectural Brief. However, reports say that centre users show a high level of satisfaction, so the financial investment made for this building will have a positive impact on users in the long term. By validating a design approach that emphasises the quality of architectural space, good design justifies a "forgiveness factor" as it has been indicated for the technical problems detected at Maggie's Dundee (Stevenson and Humphris, 2007).

To achieve a good level of design, Maggie's architects put in a lot of effort, dedication and hours of work. As Jasmin Sohi said "architects probably work harder on Maggie's projects. I put 50% more time in. I mean, we killed ourselves, but we enjoyed doing it" (*de Rijke and Sohi, 17.12.2018*). In both 'scale' and 'visibility', a commission for a Maggie's centre might be compared to that for the Serpentine Pavilion in London or a Pavilion at the Venice Biennale; the commission will eventually become a highlight in the architect's career. However, in the case of the Maggie's centre, it will not be a highlight for the press or for the architect's ego, but for having managed to produce, through the architecture and a strong sense of humanity, a positive psychological effect on people with cancer (*Tagliabue, 19.11.2018*).

As Bjørg Aabø (Snøhetta) said: 'This project is able to bring out the best that is in you as an architect'.

But how does Maggie's manage to push architects to go beyond themselves and make users extremely satisfied by enhancing their wellbeing? As explained in Chapter 4, the 'Client–Architect–User' triad is a key feature of the architectural practice, a dialogue in which, through the brief, the client instructs and collaborates with the architect who will produce a building for the benefit of users. In the case of the Maggie's centre, as a 'superb' product of Maggie's Triad, the co-clients direct the architects towards this perspective by using the Architectural Brief which, describing the emotional and sensory states that the building should evoke in its users, defies the automatic professional response.

Going back and listening to the interviews with the architects, I realised that by interpreting the emotional demands of Maggie's Brief and applying them to their projects, and bringing their own personal experiences into them, the architects were prompted to design a building that managed to evoke sensory and emotional states in users. In short, given the very difficult challenge that the co-clients have launched, only by letting themselves be 'emotionally involved' will Maggie's architects be able to provide the correct answer, responding to the Brief and going beyond it and themselves. It is at this level that a dialogue is established between architects and users which, on the one hand, sensitises the architect towards the users and, on the other, assigns a role to the users within Maggie's Triad. In this, aware of the emotions and feelings activated in them by the architect, Maggie's users undertake to pass them on to the users of other healthcare facilities, helping them to recognise an architecture that makes them feel good, becoming active subjects in the design process of the Maggie's centre.

In order for Maggie's way of 'Commissioning the Architecture' to become a reference model that can be applied to other realities, as mentioned, the relationship of the triad must be harmonious and balanced and each of the three protagonists must contribute to guaranteeing the final success of the project. To verify that Maggie's Triad is in balance, I thought of representing it graphically, observing that the main components (Co-Clients, Architect, Users), governed by the Architectural Brief and supported by the Builder, form a stable structure. In fact, the triangular scheme on the next page shows how, under each of the three vertices, a more complex development of equally contributing sub-components—all those seen so far in this book—unfold, giving rise to Maggie's paradigm for a new 'Commissioning of Architecture'. Components and sub-components can be summarised as follows (Figure 7.1):

1 Co-Clients or Client-expert (supported by the Builder who share the belief "design is a form of care") who commission the architect to design a building based on the Architectural Brief (emotional, rooted in the Benedictine 'Rule', in which architecture, programme, and values coincide) and the Support Programme, open and flexible, which promotes the motto 'empower the patient' (rooted in the Greek *Therapeutikós*, i.e. the compassioned coexistence of therapeutes and invalids).

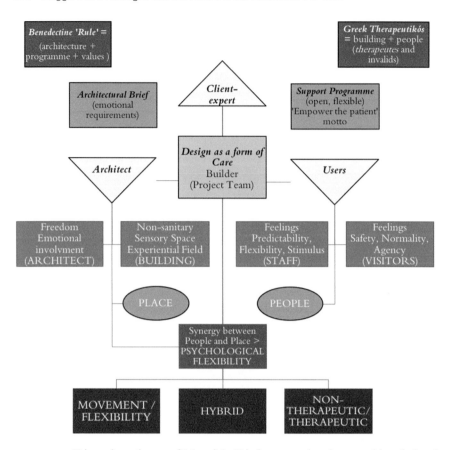

FIGURE 7.1 Triangular scheme of Maggie's Triad system showing a stable relational structure.

2 Architect who creates a building delivered through the Builder by applying the Architectural Brief to his/her own project conceived with freedom and triggered by emotional involvement, resulting devoid of signs of sanitary architecture, characterised by a sensory space and an experiential field.

3 Users (Staff and Visitors) solicited by the Support Programme offered by the Staff (*people*) who, in synergy with the building (*place*), guarantee *stimulus, predictability, flexibility* that lead to feelings of *safety, normality* and *agency*, which enable Psychological Flexibility in Visitors, strenghtened by movement, the hybrid and non-therapeutic/therapeutic nature of the therapeutic environment.

As I did in Chapter 4, in the following sections I will examine each of the components of Maggie's Triad system, this time based on the emotional involvement of the architects and their way of communicating with users. Even if the architect does not have a direct dialogue with them, by adopting a phenomenological approach, almost a 'mental transfusion', an 'I–in–them', the architect manages to convey a message of humanity to the users. In addition to addressing the architects' suggestions—which

I pass on to potential designers of future projects—, I will report inputs from the co-clients and formulate a taxonomy of feelings experienced by Maggie's users based on the therapeutic effects released by the building. Indeed, users of other healthcare facilities should be aware of this, just as new clients should take it in consideration when writing a new brief. With everyone contributing equally to the design process of the Maggie's centre, Maggie's Triad is becoming the new paradigm of the Architecture of Care.

Co-Clients (and Builder) and The Architectural Brief

> *We identify ourselves in different ways and one of them is by our environment.*
> (Architectural Brief, 2007, p. 1)

The way Maggie's co-clients approach and appoint an architect, and the relationship that is then established, differs from what usually happens in professional practice. Having discussed this topic with some architects I interviewed, and being an architect myself, I can say with certainty that often in architecture this relationship is a disconnection that leads to a considerable waste of energy and resources, manifesting a problem in the profession. In this sense, Maggie's is an exception: with a great sense of responsibility and commitment on both sides, in an atmosphere of collaboration, the relationship between co-clients and architect is always one of encouragement 'to go beyond themselves' with the ultimate goal of benefiting the users. To this end, even if external to the Triad but fundamental for the *project team*, the relationship with the builder and the people who work around him is even more important.

> At Maggie's, every single project has this 'team mentality'. So, the trickle-down effect from the visitor being the most important comes all the way through the supply chain. Even to the subcontractors on site. They know who they're delivering for and this is how we achieve the quality of the buildings that we have done.
> (*Maggie's@Salus, 2021*)

From a construction point of view, Maggie's suggests relying on builders who share the belief "design is a form of care". Therefore, the *project team* of a future centre must involve managers (project leaders, contractors, consultants) who are aware of working for a charity and who must be ready to give their maximum availability, but who consider it a privilege to work on these projects, because, in the end, they will have done something very special for Maggie's users.

> Maggie's has very few rules that they must absolutely be adhere to. This means that there is an element of flexibility for the designers and the trades people to learn and integrate with each other. Which means that they can ultimately deliver the right thing exceptionally; and that is something that we were very passionate about, instilling that understanding on the site, from the trades people and through the design team, that they are all integral parts

of this process, that they are all accountable and responsible for making sure that this particular instance of what Maggie's do is perfect for what it needs to do.

(Special Projects Sir Robert McAlpine@Salus, 2021)

In regard to the choice of the architect, who must be mature—"which does not mean old" (*Lee, 18.05.2019*)—despite the fact that in recent times many new architects have offered to design a Maggie's centre, so far the relationship between the co-clients and the architect has always begun on the initiative of the co-clients. As already explained, in the past, many of Maggie's architects were friends or former students of Charles Jencks, some of whom were already well-known, or rose to fame later thanks also to their design for Maggie's. In addition to the fact that visibility has helped bring many donors to the organisation, notoriety mostly means skill, which is what has helped Maggie's most to grow. But how is this result achieved? What is the recipe for its success?

According to the co-clients Laura Lee and Marcia Blakenham, the ingredients for success concern a few albeit crucial points: a good brief, a good client, clear ideas, and not too many outsiders, keeping the architects focused on the project and on the final goal which is to make people feel well, the ultimate goal of architecture. As mentioned, hospitals usually assemble a committee composed of many members, which plays the role of the client and, by way of a brief, appoints the architect. This brief is usually heterogeneous, made up of too diversified requests from each member of the committee, to which the architects struggle to respond to. "Hence, hospitals must first of all write a good Brief and have it handled by only a couple of design managers" (*Lee, 18.05.2019*). By keeping the commissioning management in the hands of two or three people at most, using a clear and concise Brief, to ensure that the architect achieves the final goal in a linear way, the client must keep the architect away from politics or any sponsors' requests and make sure that architects are not 'distracted' in trying to please everyone. This means that the architect must be willing to listen and the client must not impose too many instructions.

> And I think there is another thing that can influence, that is how to brief, how to be a better client, which is actually a hard work. Don't give people too many assumptions or constrains, because every time you say you want something, we often just want what we already know. There are architects who are creative thinkers and then there are architects who just got an idea already. By saying what you want, you inhibit their creativity.
>
> *(Lee, 18.05.2019)*

Since creativity also arise from the architect's freedom in interpreting the Architectural Brief and since, as already mentioned, it is not the co-clients' goal to theorise and make "assumptions on how the person entering the door must feel" co-clients work with the architect is in the name of freedom. As explained previously, this freedom comes from the concise Brief which is, on the one hand, a set of rooms, and on the other, a "very British and inhibited 'not much said'" (*Gough, 16.05.2018*). Yet, the "not much said" on its own constitutes the way the co-clients achieve their goal: paradoxically, without asking, but with a lot of guidance, the co-clients will obtain from the architect the project they want. "Yes, the less you give and the more they think for themselves" (*Lee, 18.05.2019*).

According to the co-clients, this is the best, indeed, the only way to manage the relationship because, by doing so, the project for the building will reflect both the client's and the architect's aspirations, thus ultimately allowing the users to find their own way. In the "white space between the lines", the architect will garner a great deal of references that will be transferred into the design of the building, which will allow emotions and feelings in the users. In its essentiality, the Architectural Brief, open and flexible to any interpretation, is the hidden recipe for Maggie's success.

Architects and Their Emotional Involvement (and Design Top-Tips)

> I don't think there's any of us who are not touched in some way by the impact of cancer. I had an uncle who died at 30 years old from stomach cancer, and I remember as a child experiencing that. So, you are exposed to it, you understand, I think most of us understand what the impact is. So, in that sense it's a common understanding.
>
> (*Harbour, 12.07.2018*)

From the interviews I had with Maggie's architects, focused on how they interpreted and applied the Architectural Brief to their project, it emerged that, in one way or another, cancer has touched their lives. This fact revealed something fundamental: Maggie's architects were all emotionally involved. In addition to the experience of having contributed to Maggie's mission, what the architects have in common is, in fact, an emotional involvement and, consequently, the ability to put people with cancer at the centre of the process. As Frank Gehry told me, moved by remembering Maggie, "the building needs humanity and respect, and generosity; it needs generosity to the patients". He believes whole point of this building is to forget why you are there. "So, the building shouldn't be about the architecture, it should be about them. And if it is in that way, finally, the architecture is better anyway" (*Gehry, 18.06.2018*). According to Richard Murphy—who has always been much more interested in people than in symbols—our goal must be to pursue "humanity in architecture, of how people interact with spaces and with each other and how buildings can make that possible" (*Murphy, 11.06.2018*).

It is true that each of us, even remotely, may have been involved in a cancer experience, but for an architect dealing with a theme that has to do with the struggle between the life and death of others is not an easy task to execute and complete successfully.

it's a serious project and it's brought out the best in architects, our wonderful profession, which is of course, [like medicine] ideal and utopian in every way.

(Jencks, 2019, 5:20)

As Jencks explains, Maggie's architects are called to reflect on the relationship between Architecture and Health, which, as seen in the Introduction, is an ancient theme and for which their emotional involvement is central. As mentioned, this involvement pushes the architects—who fully understand the mental state of their users—to go beyond the expected response to the client's call, a fact that clearly emerged when seeing the amount of the architects' archive material produced during the design process: the large number of sketches, watercolours, drawings, collages, photomontages and models at all possible scales and techniques showed the extra effort each architect put into their Maggie's centre, a project very small in size, but enormous in human content.

Of course, it's not a project you make money from. It's a project you do out of love. Architecture is the art of creating special places, it's not a business, it's not a commercial enterprise, it's an enterprise aimed at elevating the place.

(*McVoy, 26.05.2018*)

In addition to commitment and dedication, the small building requires the ability to release a psychological impact. As Chris McVoy states, every good architect understands that space can have a positive impact on your wellbeing. During the design process, emotional involvement leads architects to improve ideas and create solutions so innovative they can be defined "architectural inventions". For example, Chris said that at Maggie's Barts the idea of creating a luminous glass and making the colours move around it, in a sort of musical notation inspired by the medieval music played in the nearby church of Saint Bartholomew the Less, was for Steven Holl a way to infuse a deep meaning into the building and from it release a positive atmosphere of light and colour for people.

And we invented a new kind of glass, almost like a 21st century stained glass that has colour in grid and the light is calming, it's warming, and the colour gives that kind of positive energy, in a way. The thing about light is its energy.

(*McVoy, 26.05.2018*)

At the same time, the difficult content of the building, which touched some architects personally, led to the danger of their being more involved than they should be. In this regard, a significant example comes from the experience of Norman Foster, which I heard about from Charles Jencks. During the design phase of Maggie's Manchester (2016), and when the meetings with the co-clients took place, the discussion often shifted from architecture to human problems; they were about how people under stress would feel while having lunch in the garden or in the greenhouse surrounded by flowers and plants, or looking at nature from a garden window, or from the terrace in the sun, and so Foster insisted that there was a safe place where people could immerse themselves in nature and from where they could look at the horizon.

> The greenhouse was very much Norman's idea of creating this transition space, which allows the landscape to come into the building. Norman felt the idea of producing flowers that are grown in the garden, bringing them into the centre, was very important.
>
> (*Haylock, 12.06.2018*)

As Jencks reports, Foster's approach to creating an appropriate context for healing oscillated between problem-solving and spiritual or aesthetic issues, giving the impression that he understood the problem much more than one might expect. There is a reason for this, and its existential background is worth explaining.

> He and his late wife Wendy, who had succumbed to cancer in 1989, knew Maggie, and the four of us had met socially several times. Moreover, we had given them a brief overview of Chinese architecture when they were competing for the Hong Kong Shanghai Bank in 1979. I mention this and the fact of many personal meetings over the years because, when Norman finally addressed the question of designing a cancer caring centre, he was already highly motivated.
>
> (Jencks, 2018)

Norman and his late wife Wendy, who died of cancer in 1989, knew Maggie and Charles, the four of them meeting many times during their years of friendship. Despite this, nothing had ever emerged from the private life of Norman Foster, a world-renowned designer with a practice of 1,500 people and offices across the world. Yet, at the end of the film "How Much Does Your Building Weigh, Mr. Foster?"—a biopic produced by Spanish director and Norman's wife Elena Ocher (2010)—Foster reveals that he had a heart attack and cancer, and that he managed to fight back thanks to his willpower. This revelation was a surprise for everyone, as well as offering an unedited version of the projected image of someone who was invulnerable.

> Perhaps this reaction to a death sentence is an archetype with cancer, but it is one of the few cases where an architect has admitted or presented a personal response, and I have seen a direct connection between existential motivation and architectural commitment.
>
> (Jencks, 2018)

Maybe also because Norman Foster was born in Manchester, from the interview I had with his partner Darron Haylock, it emerged that the commitment that the entire office dedicated to Maggie's Manchester (2016) and the results achieved—as it happens for all the centres—went beyond expectations: the modification of the masterplan of the hospital, a former car park which has now become a lush garden, a light and airy space reminiscent of an aircraft hangar, the tall and thin wooden ballerina-like structure with outstretched arms which punctuates the space with skylights shaped like triangular crystals are clearly the result of the motivation behind such a humanly touching topic. All supported by a sense of sustainability of the construction, in terms of materials in respect of people's health, and of construction technology in compliance with costs.

> I think everybody felt that timber was the right material because of its bio-references, connection to nature, and the warmth that it brings. The idea was then embedded in the design when working with our engineers, employing timber effectively and efficiently to create the architecture, the building image, and using the structure to express that.
>
> *(Haylock, 12.06.2018)*

With Maggie's Manchester, RIBA Awards Winner in 2017, it clearly emerges that the existential motivation of a Maggie's architect—Norman Foster and his team—was the driving force behind the creation of this work, according to many critics "the most beautiful new building in Manchester" (Confidentials, 2016, para.14).

Other architects have been emotionally involved with cancer, not themselves personally, but family members or friends who have died of cancer. For example, Alex de Rijke lived the cancer experience through that of his girlfriend Lucy, who was hospitalised for six months at Christie's Manchester Hospital, while he, to be close to her, spent six months at the nearby Maggie's Manchester (2016). Learning a lot from his stay, Alex realised that, for example, to overcome the problem of shock when cancer patients touch metal, wooden handles were needed. So, in his Maggie's Oldham, which was almost completed at the time, he decided to change all the door handles from metal to wood. The tragedy of Lucy's illness, who died shortly after the opening and to whom Alex dedicated the building, made Maggie's Oldham (2017)—which Alex de Rijke believes is the most beautiful building he has ever designed—an existential motivation that eventually awarded Maggie's and the architect with the RIBA National Award 2018.

Benedetta Tagliabue, who designed Kálida Barcelona (2019), and who lost her husband, Enric Miralles, to brain cancer several years ago, also won an award, the 2020 Simon Architecture Prize. During our interview, she told me about the last days she spent with Enric in a Tibetan centre (very close to Maggie's philosophy) located in Houston, near the hospital where he was hospitalised. Many years later, when her name was suggested for the job by a group of energetic women who wanted to build a Maggie's centre in Barcelona, Benedetta gladly accepted because she felt prepared, not because of any particular scientific knowledge of healing architecture, but because of her personal experience lived with her husband's cancer, which had meant learning in advance all that she needed to know.

So, I remember a big thing, 'oh now let's sit here and we don't think for an hour'. It was so important, you know? You just say okay, this hour is okay, because maybe terrible things will happen soon, but now you can stay very well. So, these little exercises are so fundamental and a place like Maggie's can give that and can give you this time, because you don't know how long it will be, but it's a nice time and at a moment like that, this is so fundamental.

(Tagliabue, 19.11.2018)

As suggested by Annemans et al. (2012), for an architect, completing a successful healthcare building "would be impossible without a client who is actually strong enough to stand up to get the project realised the way it is designed" (2012, p. 7). At the same time, concerned with satisfying their users, Maggie's architects will 'go beyond themselves' in applying the Architectural Brief because they are emotionally involved. Because Maggie's architects were deeply affected by this experience, gaining knowledge and wisdom, I conclude this section with their design top-tips that will help other architects design future healthcare facilities (Table 7.2).

TABLE 7.2 Design Top Tips for future architects

	Maggie Architects Interviewed in 2018	*Design Top Tips for future architects*
1	Alex de Rijke/Jasmin Sohi (dRMM) (2 May/17 Dec)	Make a clear statement of the relationship between Architecture and Health
2	Piers Gough (CZWG) (15 May)	A good Architectural Brief is blind. Read between the lines
3	Ellen van Loon (OMA) (16 May)	Provide a 'menu' of spaces to accommodate people's mood
4	Chris McVoy (SHA) (26 May)	Use light as a 'material' to infuse energy
5	Richard Murphy (RMA) (18 June)	Provide habitable spaces where people can isolate themselves and still feel part of the scene
6	Frank Gehry (Gehry Partners) (23 June)	Don't think of architecture with a capital A. Give your building humanity, respect, and generosity
7	Wendy James (James&Garber) (30 June)	Clarity in the way you organise space makes a clear mind
8	Darron Haylock (Foster+Partners) (12 July)	Employ material effectively and efficiently
9	Ivan Harbour (RSHP) (20 July)	Provide continuity of space to obtain an evolving experience
10	David Page (Page\Park) (1 October)	Don't apply scientific knowledge, use your intuition
11	Bjørg Aabø (Snøhetta) (2 November)	Welcome people with a skylight and make them feel at home with a cup of tea
12	Benedetta Tagliabue (EMBT) (19 November)	Make people and the hospital proud of their healthcare facility

Users and Feelings (Enabled by Building Effects)

During interviews with the visitors of the three centres of my ethnographic work (Maggie's Dundee, Maggie's Oldham and Maggie's Barts), I learned many personal stories that people told me expressing different emotions and feelings. In general, even just mentioning the word 'cancer' generates bad emotions. At Maggie's, however, anything negative, difficult to bear when you don't have a favourable environment, as said several times, becomes tolerable. By working in synergy with Maggie's programme and applying the emotional requests of the Architectural Brief (2015), architects have been able to charge their buildings with therapeutic effects, of which the users are fully aware.

> So, these architects get a brief from Maggie's and they start even getting the germ of an idea. They know what it's for. So, they know the whole cancer thing. So, it must influence the way they design a building, right? So, what's therapeutic really comes in here as well.
>
> (*Follow-up Dundee*)

In designing their buildings, Maggie's architects adopted very different design approaches. Using the plans of the 18 buildings at the time, and analysing them according to the criteria of 'entry', 'circulation' and 'relationship with the landscape', in his book *The Architecture of Hope* (2015, pp. 32–36), Charles Jencks compared the buildings, cataloguing them by typology ranging from 'pinwheel', to 'spiral pinwheel', 'donut', 'straight', 'blob', 'L-shape'. Based on this precedent, I thought of adding a new criterion to the taxonomy of buildings: that of emotions and feelings. Indeed, in addition to typology and function, architecture should be measured and classified according to the emotions and feelings it arouses in people. For this reason, during my ethnographic work, I explored a taxonomy of feelings generated in users by the psychological effects released by buildings. Recalling that between the lines the Architectural Brief hides its secrets, analysing it one last time in depth, I managed to uncover the effects that the building releases: *impact*, *presence*, *memory*, which are the same ones that any good architecture should release. The surprising aspect about Maggie's Brief (2015) is that it describes them clearly.

> *Impact*
> Maggie's centres can and should look (and feel) bold and self-confident, as well as inviting and safe. They must look and feel joyous; they must have zest as well as calm. The impression they must give is 'I can imagine feeling different here'.
>
> (p. 6)

Described throughout the Architectural Brief, *impact* is the most important of the three effects because it must persuade the vulnerable and frightened visitor to enter the building. From afar it must attract and intrigue; closely it must encourage and invite. In this invitation, the building should tell new visitors that the experience that awaits them will make such a difference in their lives that, once they leave, they will never be the same person again.

Presence
These buildings and gardens, the way they are furnished, the art on the walls or in the garden, are designed to help people draw on strengths they may think they no longer have. (…) We ask spaces in our buildings and gardens to allow the people who use them to take charge of how they want to use them. We encourage them to make choices.

(p. 6)

In the Architectural Brief there are many possible descriptions of *presence*. The way it is meant in the description above is 'being there for them'. Like an old friend, the Maggie's centre is predictable and reliable, always bright even when it's raining outside, and has always something new to tell which is why visitors, even if they know the building by now, never get tired of coming. In the puzzle of effects, the *presence* of the building also means adaptability and flexibility, accommodating people's moods.

Memory
We want Maggie's to shelter you but to be open to the outside world, to encourage you to look out. (…) Sheltered inside, it helps to be reminded by a seasonal and changing scene outside, that you are still part of a living world.

(pp. 6–7)

The idea that *memory* of a place exists, which means that there is an image imprinted on our mind to hold on to in difficult moments, is enhanced by the interaction with nature, which Maggie's generously offers. As already explained in Chapter 5, mindful of the view from the first floor of Maggie's Dundee, my participant who had a short prognosis to live (and who unfortunately is no longer with us) had the strength and serenity—thinking of her husband who would be left alone—to submit an application to open a window in her attic, just like the one at Maggie's Dundee. This view, imprinted so deeply in Anne's memory, represents the impact of architecture and the prolongation over time of the emotional bond it creates.

Each of these effects has an implicit purpose: *Impact* offers the newcomer a *change*, moving from a dead-end situation to one with perspective, restoring the joy of living; *Presence* offers visitors a *choice* of how to continue their journey while feeling free to move through the healing process at their own pace, gaining flexibility and enduring suffering; *Memory*, creates in the veteran visitor an image to remember and rely on in difficult moments, fuelling the *hope* of a future to be planned.

In an attempt to convey the emotions and feelings generated in them by the effects released by the building, Maggie's users dialogue with users of other health facilities, helping them to recognise an architecture that makes you feel good, while earning a place in the Triad.

Feelings aroused by Impact

> When I was in the hospital after my operation, my ward looked down over the Tay. And it was so beautiful. And I could see Maggie's, the roof and the building, and people coming and going, and I knew, I knew it was to do with cancer, but I didn't really know what the ethos was, and I decided to come.
>
> (Move-along _ no.4 Dundee)

> I came one day, and there was a lot of people, I noticed. I must have arrived at the same time as many others and I thought 'No, I can't deal with this'. I went home and I did the same thing again, the following day. So, I came back on the following Monday and it was quiet and calm, and I couldn't see people. This time, I went in, and somebody almost grabbed me and said 'Hello. Come on in and have a look around'. And I think the entrance—because you can't actually see a lot from the entrance—seemed calm rather than, when you go into a hospital where there are people at reception. There's none of that here, it's calm.
>
> (Move-along_no.4 Oldham)

> Only then I realised where it was. I had to work it out because it's different, it melts in. I think it's really beautifully done, and somehow, I really noticed it, and I was bit apprehensive in coming in, where to start, I didn't know quite where to go, but immediately, while I was coming in, the staff came to say hello. So that was my first encounter. I couldn't believe it, astonished by everything.
>
> (Focus-group Barts)

The feelings generated in the users by the *Impact* of the building and by the door—as we know the most important element in this phase—can vary depending on the person; moreover, people can make several attempts before entering. So, in addition to eliciting familiarity and welcome, the *Impact* of the building must be sufficiently reassuring to always be able to try again.

Feelings aroused by Presence

> It's a sanctuary because it's away from the hospital but connected to life. At the beginning I thought this was a place where you go at the end, and I didn't realise it was about living rather than dying. There is a feeling of total tranquillity, a church quality, and safety.
>
> (Move-along_no.4 Dundee)

> I think this is a safe environment where you can talk to people. You speak to experts on the site. And you don't feel like you're taking them away from the jobs. And it's so relaxing, and its design is so warm.
>
> (Focus-group Oldham)

And that's what's so nice about the place. You know, it's not like when you're out in the world and people are expected to talk about 'it', or they're given us stupid quotes. You don't know what you're talking about! Here, you do what you want. That's why it's safe, you don't have to talk about it, we can talk about it, you can talk about a little bit, we can talk about a lot. It's accepted, done.

(Move[sit]-along_no.6 Barts)

The feelings generated in the users by the *Presence* of the building are those of trust in being sure that 'the building is there for me' and of safety and control which lead the visitors to refer to it as a safe environment that asks for nothing in return. In reality, unbeknownst to them, with an unconventional architecture and a hybrid and contradictory nature, the building subtly encourages people to make choices.

Feelings aroused by Memory

I've had a couple of days when I felt that I didn't feel good. So, I stayed home but remembering the arts [the art therapy course] made me feel better.

(Follow-up Barts)

The feelings generated in users by the *Memory,* even on those days when they cannot go to Maggie's, comes from the idea that Maggie's exists, gives courage and hope, when they say: "I wake up in the morning, and it's [cancer] here all the time". Furthermore, knowing that, as we saw in Chapter 6, there is a biological explanation for our association of memory with place—recognition neurons are stored in the hippocampus where we also consolidate long-term memories (Williams Goldhagen, 2017)—leads us to conclude that the architecture helps to remember about our past experiences, and "hold on to the meaning, sense and emotions these experiences provided us" (Schacter, 1996, p. 5). Similarly, knowing what the feeling of *wellbeing* consists of, which at a biological level is felt when 'mind' and 'body' blend (Damasio, 1994), is essential so that visitors can recognise an architecture that makes you feel good.

Emotional experiences comprise hundreds of different factors, if not thousands of different factors. So, it's quite difficult to put your finger on one thing and say: 'you feel good'. Maybe, we know, because we know the background of this building; we know we live in an iconic building, that's even famous in the UK context. So, we know, maybe that helps, as well.

(Follow-up Dundee)

By 'knowing' how they feel—"It's just how you feel" *(Follow-up Dundee)*—Maggie's users contribute to the Maggie's centre design process, confirming their role in the Triad and the *design team*. It is at this level that, as well as with users of other facilities, they are able to communicate with architects whose efforts and talent they greatly appreciate.

I think they're trying to create something, and they strive to create something that they can plug themselves into, you know, to get that 'recharged feeling'. So, they can't all be wrong and want to create iconic buildings, because they are amazing architects in their own right. And it's their gift. And I think it's their gift back to something they can do, and that's what they want to do.

(*Follow-up Dundee*)

All these thoughts have formed a taxonomy of feelings (see the diagramme in Appendix V) which should help users of other facilities to learn the difference between a 'bad' and a 'good' space that is, to understand how to recognise an architecture that makes you feel good. As we will see in the next chapter, by adding a new criterion to the way of cataloguing buildings, the judgment based on emotions and feelings will result in the paradigm of a new way of perceiving architecture.

Looking to the Future: Applying Maggie's Model

The ultimate goal of this book is to highlight the key elements of Maggie's model in order to pass them on to architects, clients and other interested parties so that they can be applied to other healthcare and non-healthcare realities. As seen, of the three Maggie's Fundamentals to be extended to the healthcare sector, the most urgent is Maggie's Triad and its way of 'Commissioning of Architecture', whose contributors and ties enable the iterative process (commissioning a centre, supervising the construction of another and outfitting the one that is about to be completed) and the creative one that gives life to a 'superb' product. This implies the transmission of Maggie's second fundamental, the Architectural Brief or, rather, what is not written in the Brief, which corresponds to the portion of freedom of interpretation left to the architect. Similar to the Benedictine 'Rule' architecture, programme and values are concentrated in it. Contrary to the current hospital way of Commissioning of Architecture, i.e. the 'Design by Committee', the principles of Maggie's Triad—based on the Architectural Brief which serves as the heart of Maggie's entire body—trigger the paradigm shift for a new 'Commissioning of Architecture' in Healthcare (Table 7.3).

TABLE 7.3 A paradigm 'Shift' for a new 'Commissioning of Architecture'.

Current 'Commissioning of Architecture'	Future 'Commissioning of Architecture'
Fragmented Brief based on functions and rules	Concise Architectural Brief based on feelings and freedom
Design by Committee	Co-Clients (max. 2-3 people)
Specialist's scientific, technical knowledge with standardised solutions	Architect's intuitive, emotionally engaged knowledge with personalised solutions

(*Continued*)

TABLE 7.3 (Continued)

Current 'Commissioning of Architecture'	Future 'Commissioning of Architecture'
Users don't count, they feel anxiety and don't know where donations go	Users count, they judge by emotions and feelings and know where donations go
Design Committee–Architect relationship with too many requests	Co-Clients–Architect dialogue with freedom and very few requests
Design Committee–User relationship through questionnaires	Co-Clients–User dialogue through participation
Architect–User relationship through a technical POE	Architect–User dialogue during visits to the centres, through a POE based on the user-experience and on an emotional level
Professionals not interested in collaborating with each other	*Project team* totally dedicated to the cause working in close collaboration

In terms of architecture and its typology, Maggie's model has two major features that could be extended to both healthcare and non-healthcare facilities:

1 The pavilion typology, i.e. Maggie's small size compared to the big hospital. This reminds us of the myth of David and Goliath. Maggie's is David and proves victorious because he is more agile and crafty than Goliath, the gigantic hospital. Despite its small size, Maggie's succeeds in contrasting the large hospital.
2 A design devoid of sanitary architecture, where the structures of other chronic don't need it. This applies, for example, to centres for mental health, heart disease, diabetes, strokes, dementia, obesity, or multiple sclerosis (MS).

Within these two architectural features, as we will see, it is essential to transmit to healthcare structures for other chronic diseases and non-healthcare facilities all the principles and values of Maggie's philosophy (openness, personalisation, familiarity, inclusion, etc.), which highlight the person and the environment, incorporated into the Maggie's centre both through the architecture and its supporting programme, to ensure a synergy between people and place that gives rise to *flexibility*. In this, not only does the motto 'design is a form of care' count, but 'design is designed with care' does as well. The priorities are therefore reversed: taking the time to think about how people experience the building becomes more important than rushing to build large, soulless containers.

Before extending Maggie's principles, however, it is worth taking a look at what of Maggie's essence and where has already been exported. Indeed, if in the British practice of healthcare architecture the influence of Maggie's model has not yet been sufficiently successful, in the rest of the world something has begun to move. During my interview with Ellen von Loon, author of Maggie's Glasgow (2011), for example, I learned that in Denmark and Holland Maggie's model has already been applied to large hospitals, where not being able afford to build a real Maggie's centre, they have installed specific units for psychological support within the oncology department.

Two other examples of healthcare buildings inspired by Maggie's philosophy are the Centre for Cancer and Health in central Copenhagen and the Verbeeten Institute in the Netherlands a cancer treatment centre with radiotherapy. The first one, designed by NORD Architects—the designers of the first version of Maggie's Forth Valley (2017)—unlike Maggie's, is large (1,800 m²), but like Maggie's, it is non-clinical. Featuring the same ethical and design principles, it offers a relaxed, homely space where cancer patients and their families can receive counselling and rehabilitation through sun terraces, gardens and even a climbing wall that encourages movement. The second one, designed by EGM architecten, unlike Maggie's, is clinical, but like Maggie's, is personalised based on the patients and their experience. Here the spaces, full of natural light that overlook the surrounding natural environment, allow effects similar to those released by the Maggie's centre. In this case, patients and staff were directly involved in the design process and, thanks to their synergistic contribution, feel a sense of ownership and belonging to a community. These two examples, whose therapeutic environment is revealed in the feelings experienced by people, demonstrate that Maggie's seed can take root and begin to have effects in other environments as well.

To Healthcare

While Laura Lee is working towards the goal of building a Maggie's centre next to each of the' 60 oncology units in British hospitals, Charles Jencks has always talked about applying the Maggie's model to structures of other chronic diseases, that is, those for which someone does not die, but continues to live, albeit with certain limits. Some of the facilities that might look to Maggie's as a role model are, for example, those for the care of heart disease, diabetes, stroke, dementia, obesity, osteoporosis, and multiple sclerosis (Jencks, 2017). During my ethnographic work, I met people with cancer who also had other diseases, such as multiple sclerosis (MS). From these visitors I learned that in healthcare, in terms of available funds for research, care and treatment, cancer is at the top of the list, while MS is probably at the bottom.

> So, I have cancer this year, unfortunately, but also I have MS that was diagnosed in 2007. The reason I bring this up is I cannot believe the difference in care and treatment. It's like different planets, 100%. I have been diagnosed with cancer here, this year, but just in terms of treatment and care, people with cancer are given this. Unbelievable. The thing is, with MS, there are no resources, they don't do anything. Also, you know, if you are diagnosed with a chronic disease or Parkinson's, the sense of isolation is huge.
>
> (*Focus-group Barts*)

This highlights another fact and that is that it is not just a matter of applying the principles of a model to a project for a centre for dementia or other diseases, but that the entire charitable operation must have strong practical basis and be focused and dedicated, for free or almost, to cooperate.

Among chronic diseases, dementia is the one that requires special care and precautions. In studying Níall McLaughlin's research on dementia (Losing_myself, 2016), I realised that while Maggie's offers *stimulus, involvement, familiarity* and more, other facilities often don't, and sometimes intentionally so. For example, there is a common belief that for Alzheimer's patients, continuing to walk in the same direction, in circles, is a good thing. However, Sabina Brennan (2015)—already met in Chapters 3, 4 and 5—explains that walking in a ring only serves to facilitate the work of the staff who will have less difficulty controlling patients, 'safer' if they continue to walk in circles.

> And it seems to me that buildings like these are designed around the functions that the staff have to partake in, and there's no consideration about these older people having a life, and frequently, their activities are based around 'you come, sit down and watch this'. An extremely passive model.
>
> (Brennan, 2015, 43:50)

In addition to stating that the building is designed to facilitate the work of the staff at the expense of unstimulated and moreover segregated patients, as seen in Chapter 3, Brennan implies that the misinformation provided to the architect—passed off as a building requirement for this type of pathology—will lead to the wrong architectural design. "The problem is, you've being asked to build buildings that are addressing the wrong people's needs" (Brennan, 2015, 46:38).

In the same interview, Brennan explains that with dementia we fear losing *independence* and *memory*, but argues that we can counteract this loss by designing buildings that simplify our lives, prolong independence and alleviate memory loss. Furthermore, to compensate for the lack of stimuli and help the elderly adapt to the new situation, Brennan argues that design can intervene through the *personalisation* of spaces, offering an environment that recalls the comfort of a home. As already seen in Chapter 4, in fact, new residents will always try to recreate their home in an environment that they do not recognise as their own, and to which they don't feel they belong. Thanks to design, however, they could "recreate" familiar spaces from the past in the current space (Brennan, 2015).

This brings us back to the last fundamental, Maggie's *Therapeutikós* from Chapter 4, which promotes a human-centred design thinking that results in 'inclusiveness', a 'home feel' and a 'sense of value'. Since *unfamiliarity* and *depersonalisation* represent the biggest flaw in the healthcare sector,—along with overly staff-oriented design to the detriment of patients,—only by creating an engaging, familiar and stimulating environment—and only by placing the right demands on architects—will it be possible to promote the physical and emotional *wellbeing* of people in other chronic disease facilities by "making these places seem like normal worlds" (Brennan, 2015, 46:54).

To Non-Healthcare

Having extended the basic principles of Maggie's model to other healthcare facilities, knowing by now what a 'therapeutic environment' means and how to improve people's wellbeing, since *wellbeing* goes beyond the healthcare context, I propose to extend to non-healthcare facilities what would ideally make any building therapeutic: *flexibility*. As already pointed out by Ellen von Loon (*15.05.2018*), the design of a therapeutic environment implies a 'menu' of spaces. Because today it is difficult to predict how people feel tomorrow, and because every day is different, it is important to provide a 'shell' under which everyone can find the right place suited to their feelings.

> We just have to make a 'shell' that fits the best with your state of mind, in that particular moment. So, it needs quite different shades, because nobody can guess how you might feel.
>
> (*van Loon, 15.05.2018*)

Offering *flexibility* in community centres, such as care homes for the elderly and some types of educational facilities for people with special needs, would help these people respond effectively to their different social conformations. As we saw in the previous section, the design choice to facilitate the staff to the detriment of the residents creates distance between them, lowering the 'sense of community'; indeed, in an environment that does not offer flexibility in meeting users' needs, it is difficult to "feel at home" (Brennan, 2015).

For Sabina Brennan the concept of *flexibility* is very similar to that of Ellen van Loon: an architectural 'canvas' under which everyone can create their own space (2015). And since, as we know, people are different from one another, enabling a personalised experience is the key to *wellbeing* and *happiness*.

> So, obviously, what makes us happy is entirely different. To answer your question, if *happiness* is somewhat associated with a personal life aspect, is it that the architect creates a canvas that can be manipulated in segments, not a canvas that is manipulated all the time in all different ways, but a canvas that at least you're never going to please everybody, but we can still be grouped? Isn't that the architects' job in this instance is to facilitate a personalisation of portions of space, that may have to change over time, depending on the profile of residence?
>
> (Brennan, 2015, 40:50)

Extending Maggie's model to types of non-healthcare settings, offering people—who sometimes want to be very sociable and other times much more introverted—the *flexibility* of a 'shell' or a 'canvas' that adapts to states of different moods and emotions, means guaranteeing them a personalised space, which translates into a 'feeling at home', which is ultimately the recipe for *happiness* (Brennan, 2015).

Maggie's Hospital

> I think there is something that worries me about the Maggie's centre, it's not the Maggie's centre's fault, but I'm thinking to myself, well, because they're

a little 'gatehouse of humanity', sitting with a huge horrible hospital behind them, is that letting them off the hook? You know, is it saying well this is just a machine I have to go through, and you go and get your dose of humanity when you go to the Maggie's Centre? I said to Laura several times, I think it would be really interesting if we had a Maggie's hospital. And demonstrate how to design a hospital, because that's the thing that would make the big difference, I think. I might have done that in Belfast for a mental hospital. So, I've come up with a very revolutionary plan, which might change how people design mental hospitals, might. It's quite interesting actually. We need a Maggie's Hospital. It would be an interesting thing to do.

(*Murphy, 01.06.2018*)

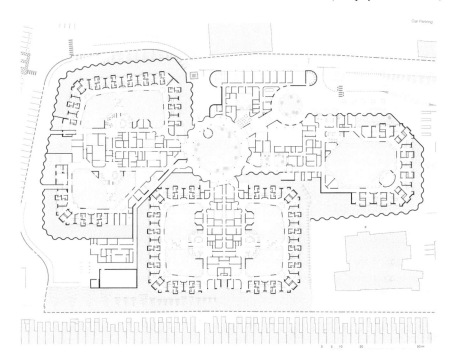

FIGURE 7.2   Ground floor plan of Acute Mental Health Facility, City Hospital, Belfast (2019) designed by Richard Murphy Architects in association with RPP Architects (Drawings Courtesy of Richard Murphy Architects).

During my interview with Richard Murphy, what emerged was the idea of bringing Maggie's embryo to a hospital, with all the characteristics of a Maggie's centre, except the attribute of being 'non-clinical'. What pushed the architect of the first Maggie's centre, Maggie's Edinburg (1996), to talk about the difference between "this mechanistic view of the hospital with respect to the human", and put forward the idea of a Maggie's Hospital—a small hospital at a time when hospitals get bigger and bigger— is a reaction. As seen in the introduction, apart from a short period of time in the 1970s, when hospitals went back to a human scale, the subsequent trend in the UK has been to become 'gigantic'. In this, the choice to build new hospitals in the middle of nowhere, where patients can be concentrated in single building and doctors have a simplified job, has led to a net decrease in family visits. "Yes, there was no particular need to move people out there, other than a lack of imagination" (*Murphy, 01.06.2018*).

The idea would be that of the 'cottage hospital', a welcoming, friendly environment where one can enter freely and, ideally, where everyone knows each other, and staff and patients look in the same direction. Just like at Maggie's, the architecture would be open, without enclosed corridors and always in contact with nature, "as hospitals once were". Farsighted and determined, as per his quote, Murphy has already applied these principles in the Acute Mental Health Facility (2019), at the City Hospital, Belfast which I visited in May 2023, leaving me struck by how the essence of the Maggie's centre was already present and had already taken root there. And since the results turned out to be excellent, Murphy's idea for a Maggie's hospital has already been revived in other projects, demonstrating that it is possible to design a hospital on a human scale (Figure 7.2).

> I mean, it is all about scale, really, and that's the problem. [...] I think it's a real shame, because a cottage hospital was a nice friendly place where people can drop in and you knew the nurses, you knew the doctors and it was a nice community centre, really.
>
> (*Murphy, 01.06.2018*)

If Murphy succeeded in his undertaking in Belfast (but his hospital other new projects are on their way), in general it seems unthinkable for the NHS stakeholders to distance themselves from the hospital as it is and go back to the small scale because there are too many factors in the design of a hospital far from the rationale of the 'ideal place', including huge budgets and veteran specialists who have very specific visions and ways of how they want to do things. Although Maggie's architects, known for their unconventional architecture, do not meet the characteristics of the healthcare professionals, if a Maggie's architect were called upon to design a hospital, it could bring about a very significant change in healthcare architecture.

> I think the problem is that we wouldn't be invited to do a hospital, because architecture is considered by the people who procure hospitals to be too particular, or too extreme, or whatever, too unconventional. But I think if we were to get to do a hospital, we could make a very significant change to what healthcare architecture looks like. I don't think it would be that difficult.
>
> (*de Rijke, 17.12.2018*)

According to Jasmin Sohi and Alex de Rijke, "because a capable architect always gets more out of a difficult situation, that is when he is challenged" (*17.12.2018*) it would not even be a problem of scale, but only of type of client. Proof of this would be the fact that, if Laura Lee were a hospital commissioner, it would certainly be possible to realise the hospital architecture at any scale. As with the Maggie's centre, however, the client should be willing to listen to potential solutions and not just their own specialists who say "that's how we always do the floor" (*Sohi, 12.17.2018*). Only by addressing the problems that arise by adopting interesting and unconventional ideas, can a special building be achieved.

> But let's say Laura Lee was a commissioner of hospitals, would you agree that it would be possible to make hospital architecture at any scale, that it could still work? So, it's not about the scale then, it's just about the patronage.
>
> (*de Rijke, 17.12.2018*)

Indeed, other architects—such as Ivan Harbour (RSHP) who designed the Cancer Centre at Guy's Hospital (2016) in London or David Page (Page\Park) who created the Woodside Health Centre (2019) in Glasgow—have already been asked to build huge hospitals and even make them look like Maggie's centre. The ability to influence other realities is, in itself, one of the principles that make Maggie's a model to imitate and, ultimately, a catalyst for a paradigm shift in the Architecture of Care. Meanwhile, one of the ways Maggie's organisation is investing is to get people to take care of their health and their families before they are diagnosed with cancer. In fact, speaking of cultural change, this is certainly the most important because it means motivating visitors to lead a healthier life and not to act when it's too late. And this is another important principle to extend to other healthcare settings (Lee, 2021).

References

Annemans, M., Van Audenhove, C., Vermolen, H. and Heylighen, A. (2012) 'What Makes an Environment Healing? Users and Designer about the Maggie's Cancer Caring Centre London', in Brassett, J., Hekkert, P., Ludden, G., Malpass, M. and McDonnell, J. (eds.) *Out of Control. Proceedings of the 8th International Design and Emotion Conference*. London, September 11–14, 2012.

Brennan, S. (2015) 'Patterns of Neurons Firing'. Interview with Sabina Brennan. Interviewed by N. McLaughlin and Y. Manolopoulou for Losing Myself. http://www.losing-myself.ie/pages/patterns-neurons-firing/

Confidentials (2016) *Maggie's: Is This Manchester's Most Beautiful New Building?* 25 August. https://confidentials.com/manchester/maggies-cancer-centre-manchesters-most-beautiful-new-building

Damasio, A. (1994) *Descartes' Error: Emotion, Reason, and the Human Brain*. London: Vintage

Ferguson, M. (1980) *The Aquarian Conspiracy*. London and Henley: Routledge & Kegan Paul

Foucault, M. (1973 [1963]) *The Birth of the Clinic: An Archaeology of Medical Perception*. London and New York: Routledge

Gray, M. (2021) 'Salus European Healthcare Design 2021: Programme Launch Webinar', 28 April. https://www.salus.global/article-show/european-healthcare-design-2021-programme-launch-webinar-1

Kuhn, T. (1962) *The Structure of Scientific Revolutions*. Chicago, IL: University of Chicago Press.

Jencks, C. (2015) 'The Art of Healing: 20 Years of Maggie's Centres'. Interview with Charles Jencks. Interviewed by A. Millar for *Leaf Review*, 7 July. https://www.leading-architects.com/features/featurethe-art-of-healing-20-years-of-maggies-centres-4628788/

Jencks, C. (2019) *Architecture of Maggie's: Charles Jencks with Alex de Rijke and Benedetta Tagliabue*. Building Centre, London, 29 May. https://www.youtube.com/watch?v=BK3N-1bBwGc&ab_channel=BuildingCentre

Losing Myself - Venice Biennale Architettura (2016) http://www.niallmclaughlin.com/projects/losing-myself/

Maggie's Brief (2015) *Architectural and Landcape Brief*. https://maggies-staging.s3.amazonaws.com/media/filer_public/e0/3e/e03e8b60-ecc7-4ec7-95a1-18d9f9c4e7c9/maggies_architecturalbrief_2015.pdf

Maggie's Evidence (2015) *Maggie's Evidence-based_Programme Web Spreads*. https://maggies-staging.s3.amazonaws.com/media/filer_public/78/3e/783ef1ba-cd5b-471c-b04f-1fe25095406d/evidence-based_programme_web_spreads.pdf

Marsh, H. (2018) *Why are Hospitals so often Horrible?* Speaker for the Phil Gusack Talk at the AfH AGM at RIBA, 22 February. https://www.slideshare.net/Architectsforhealth/henry-marsh-phil-gusack-talk-at-riba-feb-2018

Ocher, E. (2010) *How Much Does Your Building Weigh Mr Foster?* 15 December. https://www.youtube.com/watch?v=1ZC9Mf5ptd4&ab_channel=Md.MarufurRahman

RIBA (2016) *Post Occupancy Evaluation and Building Performance Evaluation Primer.* https://www.architecture.com/-/media/gathercontent/post-occupancy-evaluation/additional-documents/ribapoebpeprimerpdf.pdf

RIBA, Hay, R., Bradbury, S., Dixon, D., Martindale, K., Samuel, F. and Tait, A. (2017) *RIBA Building Knowledge: Pathways to Post Occupancy Evaluation*. Reading, UK: Value of Architects. https://www.architecture.com/-/media/gathercontent/post-occupancy-evaluation/additional-documents/buildingknowledgepathwaystopoepdf.pdf

Rosenberg, M. (1986) 'An Emerging Paradigm for Landscape Architecture', *Landscape Journal*, 5(2), pp. 75–82.

Schacter, D. L. (1996) *Searching for Memory: The Brain, the Mind, and the Past*. New York: Basic Books.

Stevenson, F. and Humphris, M. (2007) *A Post Occupancy Evaluation of the Dundee Maggie's Centre*. Final Report for Sust. https://www.ads.org.uk/wp-content/uploads/4560_new-maggiecentre1.pdf

8
EPILOGUE

Moving from Healthcare to Architecture in General

Up until now, the chapters of this book have assembled a complex and layered picture of how architecture can have an impact and "therapeutic power" in the healthcare sector. In particular, the discussion is an analysis of the different aspects that define the Maggie's centre as a therapeutic environment—its dynamic spatiality, its hybrid nature and the enigmatic and paradoxical nature of its non-therapeutic/therapeutic condition—of which *flexibility* constitutes the universal definition, explaining its fundamentals—Maggie's '*Therapeutikós*', the Architectural Brief and the Triad—and revealing the sources of its intrinsic capabilities—its synergy and its phenomenology. By the will of Charles Jencks, for whom the Maggie's centre is a 'superb product', the book has finally elected it as a paradigm for healthcare structures for other chronic diseases and non-healthcare facilities, thus making a fundamental contribution to the future 'Construction of Health'.

With the intention of opening up the discourse to architecture in general, this epilogue goes further in the attempt to demonstrate the role of design and architecture in creating a therapeutic environment outside of healthcare. Considering the 'therapeutic' as a restorative environment from which anyone would benefit, if the principles extracted from the Maggie's centre work to enable *wellbeing* and *flexibility* in people with cancer and are valid, as witnessed, when applied in other healthcare and non-healthcare facilities, they would probably be effective even when applied to architecture in general, suggesting that any building, based on such principles, could be therapeutic. Early evidence of this comes from the feedback I received from the staff at the first Maggie's Glasgow the Gatehouse (2001)–now Maggie's headquarters for Scotland–who told me that when people are visiting and the kitchen is used, the way the building–no longer a healthcare

DOI: 10.4324/9781003244516-8

facility–relates to its users is always the same and continues to be experienced as a therapeutic environment. This fact, combined with having learned the personal stories of many architects, directly or indirectly involved with cancer experiences, and having verified, through the effort put into the design of their Maggie's centre, that this experience is what prompted them to 'go beyond themselves', and finally, having learned that this experience has also influenced their way of working, impacting other projects and other clients, made me think that, once the ideal conditions are created, a set of valid design principles like the ones extracted from the Maggie's centre could influence the way in which architects work in general. But how will these principles translate so that they convey the message in architecture in general that design matters to achieve *wellbeing* and generate emotions and feelings in people, which is fundamental for overcoming traumatic transitions for all human beings?

As already explained, in Kuhnian terms, a new paradigm completely changes the way people think and act. However, as it would not be an easy task to establish a new paradigm in architectural design if not by looking at the beginning of the process—working on defining design principles into teaching and learning methods in architecture schools), I propose triggering the change by looking at the end of the process, i.e. how to judge a building, entrusting users of architecture in general with the task of verifying whether or not such principles exist, involving them in a sort of an emotional post-occupancy evaluation. Since these principles generate emotions, users of architecture in general, learning from Maggie's users, will begin to judge buildings based on the effects they emit, or no longer typologically or functionally. The new way of perceiving architecture will derive from the emotions and feelings that users will experience. The new paradigm should therefore be that of a new way of perceiving architecture. If we raise the level of appreciation and teach users not to take anything for granted, but to instead be very critical in judging spaces of living, work, leisure, etc., architects and builders will begin to change the way they design and build. Much like in the 'Users and Feelings' section of Chapter 7, in which I argued that patients of healthcare facilities should learn the difference between a 'bad' space and a 'good' one in order to convey the message in architecture that design matters in facilitating *wellbeing* and generate emotions and feelings in people, I propose that users be made more responsible. With users as spokespersons, the new paradigm will become that of a new way of understanding and perceiving architecture.

A New Perception of Architecture

Man-made space can refine human feelings and perceptions.

(Tuan 1977, p. 102)

But what are the principles of the Maggie's centre that could be applied to architecture in general so that people perceive *wellbeing* and recognise the architecture that makes them feel good? As we have seen, offering therapeutic effects and continuing to arouse emotions and feelings in us, just like the archaeological site of the healing complex of Epidaurus or a quiet cloister of the Benedictine convent still do today, the architecture of the Maggie's centre is inexhaustible. *Inexhaustibility* is the principle whereby, despite having visited it several times, a place or building continues to excite and move us, even hundreds of years later and despite the circumstances having changed. Continuing to implement over time a charge that architects call 'poetics', an inexhaustible architecture must be 'elusive', unfolding over time very slowly, revealing a new secret each time we visit, inviting us to return. Surprising us every time we come back, the inexhaustible architecture makes us feel committed and involved with affect and a sense of attachment, leading us to attribute meanings and values to it. As often happens with a Maggie's centre, every time we see it, we discover something new: the building never ceases to surprise us thanks to the secrets it hides, and these secrets are contained in the architect's project (Venezia, 2010).

In this regard, thinking that one day the Maggie's centre may change its function– as happened with Maggie's Glasgow the Gatehouse which became Maggie's office for Scotland–, I asked some architects what they thought about it. They all told me that in 50 years or more, their buildings will continue to live and be used perhaps as beautiful homes or transformed into social structures for small schools or institutes for special needs, still arousing the same feeling in their users even if their function has changed. If so, how can we apply the building's ability to adapt to new uses to architecture in general so that it continues to arouse emotions and feelings? In other words, how can we apply Maggie's intrinsic principle of *flexibility*? Among the interviewees, Alex De Rijke (17.12.2018) told me that when he visited Maggie's Gartnavel, the new Maggie's Glasgow (2011), he thought that the design team led by Rem Koolhaas had been very skilled in designing a building that was 'specific' and 'universal' at the same time: the architectural rules played in the building were very common to other forms of construction; at the same time, the way they were assembled generated something new and eternal. *Universality* is the principle according to which architecture, by renewing itself and adapting to new functions, will be understood by everyone, infinitely. This made me think that, if the Maggie's centre can be adapted to any social use and be universally understood, not only healthcare and non-healthcare buildings but also buildings in architecture in general can continue to be flexible and adaptable, generating something new and eternal, through the application of the principle of *universality.*

The principles extracted from the Maggie's centre should therefore be those of easily adapting to a new use (*flexibility*), allowing anyone to understand the place (*universality*) and making people feel emotions infinitely (*inexhaustibility*). Together with those already outlined in this book, these principles form a whole to be applied to architecture in general which, if done correctly, will lead its users to experience space and architecture not only with their eyes but also with the whole body, gaining an 'embodied experience' and learning a new way of perceiving architecture. As we saw with Maggie's users, who know their buildings well and understand the contribution that architecture makes to Maggie's mission, users of architecture in general will learn to recognise in any architecture the characteristics of a therapeutic environment and to identify in it the principles extracted from the Maggie's centre. By prioritising the cardinal principle of *flexibility*, the following list aims to help users and assist architects and builders working in general to design and construct their building to be perceived as therapeutic, with the ultimate goal of influencing the design and construction process and improving the built environment.

1   *Flexibility.* Since individuals differ from each other based on backgrounds and aspirations, therefore perceiving the built environment subjectively, and since it is difficult to predict how they feel and since every day is different, by simply creating a 'menu' of spaces that adapt to people's multiple feelings, a place or building will be flexible and adaptable to the mood of the moment (*van Loon, 05.15.2018*). At Maggie's, *flexibility* is inherent in the building and represents the movement of *people* and *place* which, in synergy with each other, activates its therapeutic environment.

2   *Unconventionality.* Usually, unconventional architecture tends to be rigid and uncomfortable. However, when combined with performativity (Butler, 1993), which makes everyone 'feel like actors', the *unconventionality* of a building or place attracts attention, making users feel curious, present, and ready to retain. In this, familiarity is not excluded. As happens at Maggie's, far from being conventional, the familiar environment of the kitchen which makes you feel at home is where, every day, good humour and *joie de vivre* are transmitted.

3   *Metaphors and Hybrid.* To put it in Charles Jencks' language, a place or a building should contain many metaphors and be hybrid, enhancing architectural richness and human values. The former in giving meaning to the content (at Maggie's, for example, the tower that offers the infinite view of the landscape is a metaphor for hope), the latter in maintaining an indefinite and enigmatic character which, in art, is a canon of aesthetics. At Maggie's, metaphors and hybrid help liberate people's imagination, allowing for feelings of empowerment and uplifting emotions that make them feel valued.

4   *Openness.* Being in an open place helps to understand the place (Tuan, 1977). Openness of space combined with openness of mind leads to a feeling of agency and control, which releases empathy towards others, activating a natural chain reaction of imitation that helps people feel included. At Maggie's, thanks to the 'spatial interaction rather than walls' which allows for synergy between *people* and *place*, visitors observe and imitate each other and think that 'if others can do it, I can do it, too', triggering the therapeutic process.

5   *Continuity.* The spatial experience is transmitted to us by the continuity of the spaces that follow one another or are inside the other, with almost imperceptible passages, leading us to experience an evolving spatial experience (*Harbour, 20.07.2018*). Like in music, these passages enable a series of imperceptible sensations that first create disorientation, but then offer a sense of *wellbeing*.

By generating movement, through open views that continuously change perspectives depending on the position of the body, the force-filled space pushes the observer so that the body merges with it. As with Maggie's, thanks to the 'movement', the observer's experience, which can be understood as an interaction between perception and action, becomes an 'embodied experience'.

6 *Human Scale.* While it may seem like a presumed variable, it makes a difference in the world of architecture when it comes to 'filling' large, depersonalised containers rather than 'dressing' human beings with a 'tailor-made' building, making these relationships reflect on it. At Maggie's, bespoke spaces consisting of a well-proportioned room, a small window, a niche combined with a carpet and a lamp that allow for comfort and *wellbeing*, help to live a personalised human experience that is ultimately the recipe for happiness (Brennan, 2015).

7 *Inexhaustibility.* In the event of a change in its intended use, the architecture must continue to move us, despite the new function and the passage of time. Almost 'elusive', the inexhaustible place or building reveals itself very slowly over time, involving and surprising us every time we visit it, inviting us to return and making us develop affect and a sense of attachment. As in the case of Maggie's, the architect's secrets hidden in the project are what keeps visitors coming back and continues to arouse emotions and feelings in them.

8 *Universality.* According to the principle of universality, in 50 years, continuing to exist with another use and adapting infinitely, universal places or buildings will still be understood by everyone, arousing the same feelings in us. In a Maggie's centre, the architectural ingredients used in the building are conceived as 'specific' and 'universal': they are common to other building forms and yet, thanks to the way they have been assembled, they generate something new and eternal (*de Rijke, 17.12.2018*).

With the aim of identifying these principles in our environment and developing the ability to recognise the architecture that makes feel good, keeping in mind the psychological effects released by Maggie's buildings (*Impact, Presence, Memory*) and the taxonomy of feelings that users experience at Maggie's (Appendix V), I suggest new users keep a notebook, a sort of 'user experience manual', in which they report their emotional experiences in order to understand what in a place is 'good' or 'bad' for us (Mallgrave, 2013). Furthermore, associating memories with places, I recommend making a list of buildings or places from our past that have had an impact on us and made us feel emotions and feelings. In this experiment, since "architecture without people becomes sculpture" (Alvaro Siza, quoted in Gepshtein and Berger, 2020, 8:40) and there is no memory of a place that has not forged our identity (Williams Goldhagen, 2017), it is essential to refer to a building or place in association with human relationships, which is what enables people's "meaning of place" and "attachment to place" (Heidegger, 1971 [1954]; Relph, 1976; Mugerauer, 1994). As Charles Jencks wrote to me in an email dated 06.11.2018, we should never forget the place. "Remember: the atmosphere, the emotion, the meaning, yes, transmitted through the usual architectural means of space, light, rhythm, matter, but also meaning and relationship with the place" (*Jencks, 11.06.2018*).

Architecture as a Tool

Architecture is a social tool because, through its spaces, it creates relationships that are vital for human beings. As soon as they enter a building or a place, even if only at an intuitive level, people understand how to behave and, thanks to personalised spaces and the way the building or place organises movement, they deduce whether the environment can generate *wellbeing* and facilitate encounters. In this, thanks to the principle of *inexhaustibility*, that is, the ability to attract and involve people infinitely, architecture will ensure that people return and meet even more people; in particular, by creating immersive experiences, designed to entertain and engage people's minds, a sensory architecture favours these encounters. In this sense, in architecture in general, the Oslo Opera House (2015) designed by Snøhetta, also the designer of Maggie's Aberdeeen (2013), represents a significant example of social tool: thanks to its accessible sloping roof–a civic device open to all–people are free to climb to the top while acquiring a sense of mastery and openness, becoming more willing to interact with others. This predisposition is aided by the geographical context characterised by the Nordic light that never goes out and by a very high sky which, acting as the backdrop to the journey, accompanies people connecting them or, rather, 'projecting' them into the surrounding landscape, allowing a sense of belonging to the place and an 'embodied experience'. Already seen with Le Corbusier's *promenade architec-turale*, the movement that the roof of the Oslo Opera House creates, and with which it invites us to engage, is a movement that makes us experience, with the whole body, emotions that influence the mind but which also encourage imitation and intersubjectivity: by pinching the strings of our senses, the phenomenological power derived from the sense of openness and accessibility of the building encourages connection with others, with the sociality, which is central in the design of an architecture or an urban place that aspires to be a social tool, which will also excite us with its *beauty*.

> The Architect, by his arrangement of forms, realises an order which is a pure creation of his spirit; by forms and shapes he affects our senses to an acute degree, and provokes plastic emotions; by the relationships which he creates he wakes in us profound echoes, he gives us the measure of an order which we feel to be in accordance with that of our world, he determines the various movements of our heart and of our understanding; it is then that we experience the sense of 'beauty'.
>
> (Le Corbusier, 1931, p. 11)

And it is to the beauty of human construction–"a datum of abstract geometry", which with its order measures the infinity of nature–that we turn to in the most difficult situations, realising how, in a historical moment like this, which, as Berthoz had predicted, is "of unprecedented violence" (2000, p. 265), architecture becomes a tool of salvation and resilience. In this sense, the experience of Lodovico Barbiano di Belgiojoso (Milan, 1909–2004) told in a small book of "extraordinary architectural lesson" and reported by Dario Banaudi (2015) is a significant one. Deported to an extermination camp in Nazi Germany from where millions of people never returned, the Italian architect–part of the BBPR group that designed the Velasca Tower in Milan–managed to survive the horrors of war thanks to the architecture that had given him the ability to imagine and therefore hope. Imagining isolating himself by building around himself "a very high wall (...) with four walls that enclosed a small field (...) four walls without doors (...) a large prism of pure air", knowing how to exercise his imagination, Belgiojoso managed to abstract himself from the atrocities that occurred in Gusen where he had also learned the lesson that everyone can make their own: "everyone got used to living on hope as here one lives on one's art, one's passion" (Belgiojoso, 1999, cited in Banaudi, 2015*).

By unleashing passion and imagination, which are those emotional and cognitive activities that fuel our lives (also remembering that thanks to passion, human beings can change themselves and the world around them [Schmarsow, 1893, cited in Mallgrave, 2013], and that imagination is much broader than knowledge because it "embraces the whole world" [Einstein, 1931]), architecture is, finally, a powerful tool of reconciliation. The result of my investigation to discover the therapeutic power of the Maggie's centre–and to reunite the 'body' with the 'mind' and reconcile the 'architecture' with the 'therapeutic'–lies precisely within the capacity for synthesis of architecture. Coming from different contexts, the disciplines I investigated–Psychology, Phenomenology and Neuroscience–have as an object of interest how humankind moves in built spaces, although their arguments and points of view follow different parameters and frames of reference. Despite this, their thoughts, once intertwined, were able to answer a question in architecture. As per Piers Gough's statement that "Architecture is the absolute mother of the Arts", I suggest that this skills-exchange mindset is reflective of the 'Renaissance' spirit architecture requires, which is characterised by a broad but also detailed vision. Inherent in the very etymological meaning of 'architect'–from the Greek ἀρχιτέκτων (architéktōn) composed of ἀρχή (árche=chief) and τέκτων (técton=builder), 'first' or 'guide' to 'create' or 'build' (Merriam-Webster, 2024)–this vision makes Architecture the only discipline capable of synthesising and directing all the contributions necessary to truly improve the therapeutic value of our built environment. As Maggie's users teach, Architecture is unquestionably and universally encompassing and calls everyone to make their own contribution within their role. Consequently, both the recognition and the ability to improve our health and *wellbeing* and that of our communities lies in everyone's hands.

Remembering Two Special Maggie's Visitors

The ethnography underlying my research and this book have shown that architecture has played an important role in facilitating my *wellbeing* and meeting with the people at Maggie's with whom I experienced emotions and feelings that left indelible memories. Since both architecture and people have had an immense impact on my life, in a way that will never go away, before concluding this book, I want to remember two special visitors–both participants of mine at Maggie's Dundee whom we already met in Chapter 5–who, soon after our first encounter became close friends. Sadly, like another visitor I met, both are no longer with us. In addition to being positive and full of energy, Philly was also a fighter. That's why she survived for a couple of years despite her diagnosis thanks to her Maggie Keswick-inspired project to create a *Philly's Centre,* which no one ever built. Anne, on the other hand, who despite her short life expectancy, had wanted to make an alteration to her house and put in a window to enjoy the view during her last two years of life, was extraordinarily positive, even in helping her husband survive her loss. Unfortunately, they did not have time to see their dreams come true, but their soul and the memory of our short friendship will remain forever in the existence of architecture.

> The poetic nature of architecture is identified in the presence and the unfolding of time throughout its existence. And in its existence over time, not at a particular moment in history. Temporality, the ability to forge relationships that shape time, moving emotions, is architecture's true secret, its soul.
>
> *(Venezia, 2010, p. 40)*

References

Banaudi, D. (2015). 'L'Architettura come salvezza', in *Farecultura*, 1(8), 6 November. https://www.farecultura.net/wordpress/arte/architettura-design/873/larchitettura-come-salvezza-a-proposito-del-libro-di-lodovico-barbiano-di-belgiojoso-frammenti-di-una-vita-archinto-editore-milano1999/

Barbiano di Belgiojoso, L. (1999) *Frammenti di una vita.* Milano: Archinto editore

Berthoz, A. (2000) *The Brain's Sense of Movement.* Cambridge, MA and London: Harvard University

Butler, J. (1993) *Bodies that Matter: On the Discursive Limits of 'Sex'.* London and New York: Routledge

Einstein A. (1931) *Cosmic Religion – With Other Opinions and Aphorisms.* New York: Covici Friede

Gepshtein, S. and Berger, T. (2020) *Dynamics of Architectural Experience in the Perceptual Field*, 16 January. https://www.youtube.com/watch?v=HI7s8OhZpT4&ab_channel=AMPS

Heidegger, M. (1971 [1954]) 'Building, Dwelling, Thinking', in Hofstadter, A. (ed. and transl.) *Poetry, Language, Thought.* New York: Harper Colophon Books, pp. 1–9

Le Corbusier (1931) *Towards a New Architecture.* New York: Dover Publications

Mallgrave, H. F. (2013) *Architecture and Embodiment. The Implications of the New Sciences and Humanities for Design.* London and New York: Routledge

Merriam-Webster (2024) "Etymology of the architect". https://www.merriam-webster.com/dictionary/architect

Mugerauer, R. (1994) *Interpretations on Behalf of Place. Environmental Displacements and Alternative Responses.* Albany, NY: State University of New York Press

Relph, E. (1976) *Place and placelessness.* London: Pion

Tuan, Y.-F. (1977) *Space and Place.* Minneapolis: University of Minnesota Press

Venezia, F. (2010) *The Poetic Nature of Architecture.* Pordenone: Giavedoni editore

Williams Goldhagen, S. (2017) *Welcome to Your World: How the Built Environment Shape Our Lives.* New York: Harper Collins.

APPENDICES

I. Architectural Brief (2007)

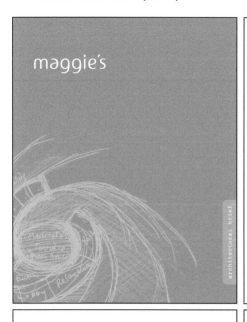

MAGGIE'S CANCER CARING CENTRES

Maggie's asks a lot of its buildings and hence of its architects. We expect the physical space to do a significant amount of our work for us.

A Maggie's Centre sets the scene for people going through a traumatic experience. They are places where people draw on strengths they may not have realised they had in order to maximise their own capacity to cope.
We need buildings where people can read themselves differently, as individuals in unusually difficult circumstances, not as patients, let alone cancer victims.

We identify ourselves in different ways and one of them is by our environment. This is why we choose architects who we think will rise to the challenge of making spaces for us which help this transition and also do apparently contradictory things.

We need our buildings to feel safe and welcoming. They need to be small, and domestic in scale. On the other hand these little buildings should not pat you on the head, patronise you by being too cosy. They should rise to the occasion, just as you, the person needing help, is having to rise to the occasion of one of the most difficult challenges any of us is likely to have to face. At the very least they should raise your spirits.

We need our buildings to recognise that the world of the hospital and a cancer diagnosis turn your personal world upside down, and that in deciding to walk through the door of a Maggie's Centre people are saying to themselves and to us: "I am adjusting to a difficult and unknown situation that I am finding hard to cope with on my own."

To a greater or lesser degree, by walking in to a Maggie's Centre people are asking how they can put their lives back together again. They are hoping for transformation.

Giving them a place to turn to which is surprising and thoughtprovoking – and even inspiring – will give them the setting and the benchmark of qualities they will need in themselves. Knowing there is a place to turn to which is special in itself makes you feel valued.

So we want the architects to think about the person who walks in the door. We also want the buildings to be interesting enough that they are a good reason to come in rather than just 'I'm not coping'. The first clinical psychologist who worked for Maggie's, Glyn Jarvis, says that working from a Maggie's Centre means that he can start a quantum leap ahead of talking to the same people in a hospital context because people have actively chosen to come in.

Maggie's Centres and the way they are designed increase the sense of connectedness between people: they are not alone in this situation and people can find ways of moving forward from the crisis of a diagnosis. The architects should be thinking about the human relationships and connections, and doing the job of helping that happen.

What we're also looking for in our architects is an attitude. We want people to deliver the brief but without preconceived ideas. We don't want to say to them: 'This is the way it is done'. We want them to open our eyes as well.

Maggie's was lucky in our architect for the first Maggie's, Richard Murphy in Edinburgh, who showed us how much a building can achieve by creating the right atmosphere.

We were also lucky to be able to draw on the close friendships of Maggie and Charles Jencks with some of the most imaginative architects working in the world today, and who have reinforced for us how much a good building can do.

We hadn't realised, until it happened, how powerful a tool it would be that each community feels so proud of its Maggie's. This works on multiple levels. Critical to the success of Maggie's is a strong feeling of ownership by the local community. It makes people feel: 'This place is wonderful and it belongs to me, and to other people in the same boat as me'. They want to come in. It provides one positive thing to look forward to in their trek to the hospital. It is critical, also, because people talk about their Maggie's. The Centres do our 'marketing' for us. Crucially, these special, unique buildings help us to raise the money we need to build them in the first place, and then to keep them running.

Our buildings are special and we chose special architects, not for some luxury add-on value, but because they are a critical component of what we do.

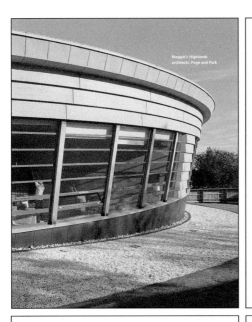

Maggie's Highlands
architects: Page and Park

THE ARCHITECTURAL BRIEF

PURPOSE OF MAGGIE'S CENTRES

To provide non-residential support and information facilities for people with cancer, and for their families and friends.

The building will offer its users a calm friendly space where each individual can decide what strategy they want to adopt to support their medical treatment and their overall welfare.

They will be able, if they so wish, to have a private conversation with the programme director or the clinical psychologist about their situation and needs.

On offer within the building will be a free programme, which will include group support, family and friends support, relaxation sessions, information access and benefits advice. (See Maggie's Centre booklets and website for programme and timetables.)

People may choose to do any of this programme or none of it. Some will want to use the Centre to have a cup of tea and a quiet pause. Others will be helped by offering volunteer services themselves, such as gardening. And others, again, will want to join support groups and actively participate.

We do not want to suggest there are better or worse ways of dealing with cancer. Any way that helps anybody going through cancer to feel better is fine, with the important proviso that any service offered in the building will be approved by the Professional Advisory Board and will be complementary and not alternative to orthodox medical treatment.

Approximate size of a Maggie's Centre is 280m²

REQUIREMENTS FOR MAGGIE'S

Entrance: obvious, welcoming, not intimidating.

Small coat-hanging/brolly space.

A welcome/sitting/information/library area, from which the layout of the rest of the building should be clear. There should be as much light as possible. There should be views out to grass/trees/sky. You should be able to see where the kitchen area is, equally the sitting room and fireplace-area (hearth & home). Maggie suggested a fish tank.

Office space for a) Centre Head and b) fundraiser/deputy. This should be easily accessible from the welcome area so that either person working at a desk can see somebody come into the Centre, in order to welcome them. Their space should be separate enough that the welcome area does not seem like an office or a reception area. There should be storage space for stationary/pamphlets/bumph accessible to the office space. Space should be allocated for a photocopier, printer, server and other office machinery. Each workstation needs a telephone, computer point and light, shelf and drawer space. As well as the main ones there should be for 5 other workstations, which can be quite small. Can we have this many work stations without it appearing to be like a huge office which dominates the Centre? They don't have to all be in one block. Somewhere for staff to hang coats.

A video-viewing and computer-link information area or bay for the use of 4 people, probably not all together, but within shouting distance of the programme director's office area, so that he/she can help if necessary.

A kitchen area, like a 'country' kitchen, with room for a large table to sit 12, which could be used for demonstrations/seminars/discussion groups. The kitchen should be relaxed and inviting enough for anybody to feel welcome to help themselves to coffee or tea. A central 'island' on which cooking demonstrations could take place would be helpful.

A large room for relaxation groups/lectures/meetings. A space sufficient to take a maximum of 14 people lying down. Storage space for relaxation/folding chairs. As much as possible, you should be able to open and shut walls (perhaps between this and welcome area/kitchen area) to have flexi-space, for more or less privacy, as occasion demands. The relaxation space should be capable of being soundproof when closed off.

Two smaller sitting/counselling room for 12 people with a fireplace or stove. This doesn't have to be very big – it makes for a friendlier atmosphere if people have to budge up a bit. Perhaps there should be dividing doors to become a second large room, although each one would need to be individually soundproof.

Two (or one if the large room can sub-divide) small rooms for counselling or therapy, preferably with big windows looking out to grass/trees/sky. They should have a bit of character and perhaps they could have sliding doors that can be left open and be inviting when not in use. They should be soundproof. One should be able to take a treatment bed, preferably facing a window.

Lavatories (probably 3) with washbasins and mirrors, and at least one that is big enough to take a chair and a bookshelf. They should not be all in a row with gaps under the doors. Private enough to have a cry.

A very small quiet space to have a rest/lie down.

Outside: garden areas and 10 parking spaces. If this is unlikely on the site, if possible make a drop-off and pick-up area and perhaps a couple of disabled spaces. We like the idea of a continuous flow between house and garden space there should be somewhere to sit, easily accessed from the kitchen. We want the garden, like the kitchen, to be an easy public space for people to share and feel refreshed by. The relationship between 'inside' and 'outside' is important. A house protects you from the 'outside'. Equally the 'outside' of a garden is a buffer to the real 'outside'. It is a place where you can feel sheltered but enjoy a bit of the kinder sides of nature. There are practical considerations about privacy, referred to later; we also want to consider how a garden can help invite you in through the door from the street (which is always a key factor) and maybe how to incorporate parking spaces without them being too intrusive.

PRACTICALITIES

We have got to run each Maggie's Centre as economically as possible without compromising what we are trying to offer. We know that any kind of complex building costs more to build, but it will have to be borne in mind, at design level, that we have a small building budget and that subsequent building maintenance and cleaning should be as cheap as possible: wood floors/ease of access/6 light fittings preferable to 56.

It might help to think of this as a 'positive' restraint, not an economic constraint, in the sense that the aim of this project is to build a modest, humane building, which will encourage and not intimidate.

OVERALL

We want to make spaces that make people feel *better* rather than *worse* (most hospitals).

Some things are obvious:

- As much light as possible.

- Important to be able to look out – and even step out – from as many 'rooms' as possible into something like a garden, a courtyard, or 'nature'. At the same time, the sitting/counselling rooms (8) and (9) should have privacy, ie if they do have doors to the outside 'rooms', passers-by shouldn't intrude.

- The interior spaces shouldn't be so open to the outside that people feel naked and unprotected. They should feel safe enough inside that they can look out and even go out if they wanted...this describes a state of mind, doesn't it?

We want to have the minimum possible 'administration office' type atmosphere. No doors with 'fundraiser' on the outside. We want the ethos and scale to be domestic. We need to think of all the aspects of hospital layouts, which reinforce 'institution' – corridors, signs, secrets, confusion – and then unpick them.

As a user of the building, we want you to approach the building, and see an obvious and enticing door. When you come in, we want the first impression to be welcoming. People may come to 'have a look', the first time.

We want Centre users to feel encouraged and not daunted: they are likely to be feeling frightened and very low anyway. We want them to have an idea of what is going on in the whole building when they come in. We want them to feel they have come into a family community in which they can participate, make their own tea or coffee, use a computer, sit down and borrow a book, even find somewhere they might have a sleep for half an hour. Things shouldn't be too perfect.

The rooms used for counselling should be completely private when they are in use; but it would be no bad thing if they could be opened up when they were not. We want users to know that they can say things in confidence and be quiet, but also be conscious that other things are going on around them that they might be interested in. For instance, they might be able to see what is going on in the kitchen but will not necessarily want to participate in the kitchen chat.

We want the building to feel like a home people wouldn't have quite dared build themselves, and which makes them feel that there is at least one positive aspect about their visit to the hospital which they may look forward to.

We want the building to make you feel, as Maggie made you feel when you had spent time with her, more buoyant, more optimistic, that life was more 'interesting' when you left the room than when you walked into. Ambitious but possible?

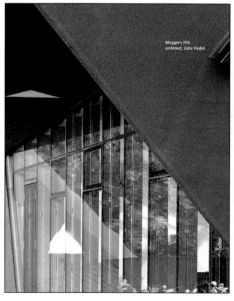

Maggie's Fife
architect: Zaha Hadid

II. Maggie's Support Programme

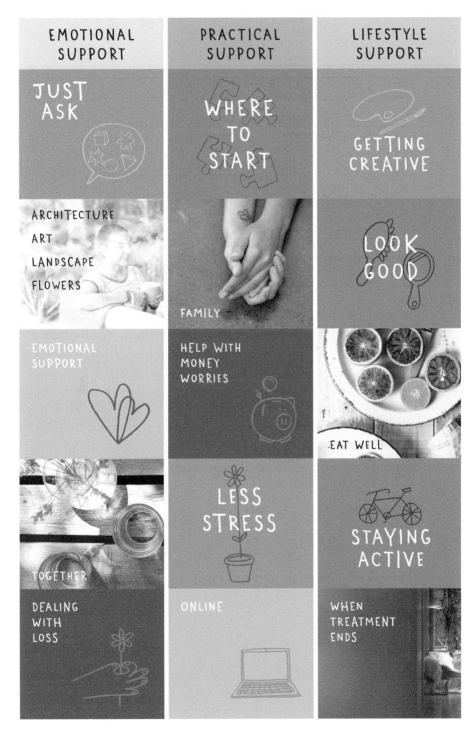

EMOTIONAL SUPPORT — PRACTICAL SUPPORT — LIFESTYLE SUPPORT

JUST ASK — WHERE TO START — GETTING CREATIVE

ARCHITECTURE / ART / LANDSCAPE / FLOWERS — FAMILY — LOOK GOOD

EMOTIONAL SUPPORT — HELP WITH MONEY WORRIES — EAT WELL

TOGETHER — LESS STRESS — STAYING ACTIVE

DEALING WITH LOSS — ONLINE — WHEN TREATMENT ENDS

III. Maggie's Map and Timeline (1996 onwards)

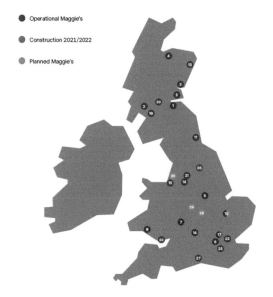

● Operational Maggie's

● Construction 2021/2022

● Planned Maggie's

EUROPE

MIDDLE EAST AND ASIA

Maggie's centres

❶ Edinburgh
❷ Glasgow
❸ Dundee
❹ Highlands
❺ Fife
❻ West London
❼ Cheltenham
❽ Nottingham
❾ Swansea
❿ Cambridge (interim)
⓫ Newcastle
⓬ Hong Kong
⓭ Aberdeen
⓮ Oxford

⓯ Wirral
⓰ Lanarkshire
⓱ Royal Free (interim)
⓲ Manchester
⓳ Tokyo
⓴ Forth Valley
㉑ Oldham
㉒ Barts
㉓ Cardiff
㉔ Barcelona
㉕ The Royal Marsden (Sutton)
㉖ Leeds
㉗ Southampton

Planned centres

⓱ Royal Free
㉘ Northampton
㉙ Coventry
㉚ Liverpool
㉛ Stavanger
㉜ Groningen

1996-2000	2001-2005	2006-2009	2010-2011	2012-2013	2014-2016	2017-2019	2021-2024

Maggie's Edinburgh, 1996

Maggie's Glasgow The Gatehouse, 2002

Maggie's Dundee, 2003

Maggie's Fife, 2006

Maggie's West London, 2008

Maggie's Cheltenham, 2010

Maggie's Glasgow Gartnavel, 2011

Maggie's Nottingham, 2011

Maggie's Sawnsea, 2011

Maggie's Newcastle, 2013

Maggie's Aberdeen, 2013

Maggie's Merseyside, 2014

Maggie's Lanarkshire, 2014

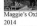

Maggie's Oxford, 2014

Maggie's Manchester, 2016

Maggie's Tokyo, 2016

Maggie's Forth Valley, 2017

Maggie's Oldham, 2017

Maggie's Barts, 2017

Kálida Barcelona, 2019

Maggie's Cardiff, 2019

Maggie's at The Royal Marsden, 2019

Maggie's Yorkshire, 2019

Maggie's Southampton, 2021

Maggie's Wirral, 2021

Maggie's at The Royal Free, 2024

Maggie's Northampton, TBC

Maggie's Coventry, TBC

IV. The Maggie's Centres Floorplans (1996 onwards)

Maggie's Edinburgh (1996)	Maggie's Glasgow-The Gatehouse (2002)	Maggie's Dundee (2003)	Maggie's Highlands (2005)	Maggie's Fife (2006)
Maggie's West London (2008)	Maggie's Cheltenham (2010)	Maggie's Glasgow Gartnavel (2011)	Maggie's Nottingham (2011)	Maggie's Swansea (2011)
11. Maggie's Newcastle (2013)	12. Maggie's Aberdeen (2013)	13. Maggie's Hong Kong (2013)	14. Maggie's Merseyside (2014)	15. Maggie's Lanarkshire (2014)
16. Maggie's Oxford (2014)	17. Maggie's Manchester (2016)	18. Maggie's Tokyo (2016)	19. Maggie's Forth Valley (2017)	20. Maggie's Oldham (2017)
21. Maggie's Barts (2017)	22. Kálida Barcelona (2019)	23. Maggie's Cardiff (2019)	24. Maggie's at The Royal Marsden (2019)	25. Maggie's Yorkshire (2019)
26. Maggie's Southampton (2021)	27. Maggie's Wirral (2021)	28. Maggie's at The Royal Free (2023)	29. Maggie's Northampton (TBC)	30. Maggie's Coventry (TBC)

V. Users' Taxonomy of Feelings

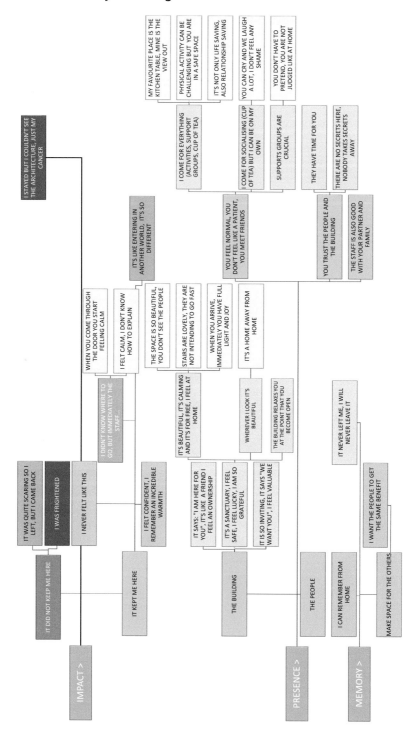

ILLUSTRATION CREDITS

Main Text

Figure 1.1 EPIDAURUS/EPIDAVROS. Hieron Asklepios/Asklepius temple/sanctuary plans 1909 map (Purchased by © 2020 Antiqua Print Gallery Ltd)

Figure 1.2A–1.2D Thomas Willis' Cerebri Anatome, 1664. Cover page, Sir Christopher Wren's drawing of the base of the brain "with the roots of the vessels cut off", pp. 25–26, *Figura Prima*, legend of the different parts of the brain (Courtesy of The Royal Society of Medicine)

Figures 2.1–2.3 Maggie's Dundee (2003) (courtesy of Maggie's), Maggie's Oldham (2017) and Maggie's Barts (2017) (©Marco Castelli Nirmal). During the day Maggie's buildings invite you to enter; at night, like lanterns, they illuminate the path of people in the darkness

Figures 2.4–2.6 Maggie's Dundee (2003) (Courtesy of Maggie's), Maggie's Barts (2017) and Maggie's Oldham (2017) (©Marco Castelli Nirmal). Entering Maggie's buildings there is a sense of projection

Unnumbered p. 33 The Maggie's centre creates movement (Maggie's Lanarkshire, 2014) (©Marco Castelli Nirmal)

Unnumbered p. 37 Maggie's centre creates a moment of disorientation (Maggie's Barts, 2017) (©Marco Castelli Nirmal)

Chapter Opener p. 46 Maggie Keswick in China (Courtesy of C. Jencks)

Figure 3.1 Charles Jencks' metal installation depicting Maggie peering into her brain in the Garden of the Six Senses at Maggie's family's Portrack House in Dumfriesshire, Scotland (Courtesy of Charles Jencks)

Figure 3.2A–3.2B Maggie's Edinburgh (1996). View of the building as it appears today and of the kitchen on the ground floor glimpsed from the upper floor (©Marco Castelli Nirmal)

Figure 3.2C–3.2D Maggie's Edinburgh (1996). View from above of the welcome area with the wooden staircase containing seating and bookcases (©Marco Castelli Nirmal)

Figure 3.3 Maggie's buildings support the staff to be present keeping an eye on visitors (Maggie's Glasgow, 2011) (©Marco Castelli Nirmal)

Figure 3.4 The open horizon view of Maggie's buildings supports Maggie's strategy of 'empowering the patient' (Maggie's Oldham, 2017) (©Marco Castelli Nirmal)

Figure 3.5 The first space that visitors arriving at Maggie's see is the kitchen. Seeing it spacious and full of people busy preparing food and drinks, newcomers immediately feel a sense of familiarity (Maggie's West London, 2008) (Courtesy of Maggie's)

Figure 3.6 Among the centres, some are more iconic than others. The iconic facade entertains and makes you smile (Maggie's Nottingham, 2011) (©Martine Hamilton Knight)

Figure 3.7 Floorplan of Maggie's Glasgow (2011) with the few functional requirements of the Architectural Brief (Courtesy of OMA)

Figure 3.8 Before entering, Maggie's buildings give you time to decide. The 'pause' space could be a simple tree trunk where you can sit and meditate (Maggie's Glasgow, 2011) (©Marco Castelli Nirmal)

Figure 3.9 The 'pause' space can also be a veranda like an American porch (Maggie's Manchester, 2016) (©Marco Castelli Nirmal)

Figure 3.10 The 'pause' space can be a series of thresholds (Maggie's West London, 2008) (©Marco Castelli Nirmal)

Figure 3.11 Maggie's welcome area/library greets visitors with colorful seats, a shelf filled with brochures and books and a notice board describing the centre's activities (Maggie's Lanarkshire, 2014) (©Marco Castelli Nirmal)

Figure 3.12 Maggie's kitchen, even when it rains, is always bright and warm (Maggie's Oldham, 2017) (©Marco Castelli Nirmal)

Figure 3.13 Different in each centre, the kitchen table can take any shape. At Maggie's Aberdeen (2017) it is oval (Courtesy of Maggie's)

Figure 3.14 Medium-sized consultation rooms can accommodate groups of up to 12 people, welcoming them with a fireplace to create a more convivial environment (Maggie's Edinburgh, 2018 addition) (©Marco Castelli Nirmal)

Figure 3.15 At Maggie's the large sitting room, furnished with comfortable armchairs, beautiful carpets, and warm light lamps transforms flexibly into a group activity room (Maggie's Barts, 2017) (©Marco Castelli Nirmal)

Figure 3.16 At Maggie's, hanging a work of art is like opening a window, it gives you a view (Maggie's Glasgow, 2011) (©Marco Castelli Nirmal)

Unnumbered p. 76 Maggie's furnishings together with architecture and nature create comfort and atmosphere (Maggie's Lanarkshire, 2014) (©Marco Castelli Nirmal)

Figure 3.17 Maggie's Gardens do much more than ordinary gardens, just like the woodland meditation place designed by Lily Jencks at Maggie's Glasgow (2011) (©Marco Castelli Nirmal)

Figure 3.18 At Maggie's Highlands (2002) the landscape is a metaphor for living with cancer told through the division of cancer cells (Courtesy of Maggie's)

Figure 3.19 Maggie's uses the greenhouse to keep people busy taking care of the land's products, a good way to lower defenses and open up to others (Maggie's Manchester, 2016) (©Marco Castelli Nirmal)

Figures 3.20–3.21 All Maggie centres offer endless views of the horizon or narrow views through small cozy nooks, over tiny gardens or up to the sky (Maggie's Glasgow, 2011) (©Marco Castelli Nirmal), (Maggie's Cardiff, 2019) (©Anthony Coleman)

Chapter Opener p. 108 Psychological Flexibility bends people's minds like reeds in the wind. View from Maggie's Dundee kitchen. (©author)

Figure 5.1A and 5.1B The *hexaflex* and *triflex* models of Psychological Flexibility (courtesy of Steven Hayes)

Figure 5.2 Maggie's kitchen helps people open-up to social interactions and 'therapeutic conversations' (Maggie's Dundee, 2003) (Courtesy of Maggie's)

Figure 5.3 Maggie's sensory space helps people be fully present (Maggie's Barts, 2017) (©Marco Castelli Nirmal)

Figure 5.4 Maggie's icons distract but also help people focus on what's important to them and act with commitment (Maggie's Oldham, 2017) (©Marco Castelli Nirmal)

Chapter Opener Maggie's phenomenology (Maggie's Glasgow, 2011) (©Marco Castelli Nirmal)

Figure 6.1A–6.1C p. 136 Maggie's Dundee (2003), plan and section diagrams of the 'hidden' structure of the experiential field. View of the oval counter wrapped in an imaginary 'bubble' of privacy enclosed underneath the intricate trussed ceiling (Drawings courtesy of Frank Gehry with diagramme by the author) (©Courtesy of Maggie's)

Figure 6.2 At Maggie's, hearing laughter is common and older visitors are not ashamed to laugh in the presence of newcomers in tears (Maggie's Dundee, 2003) (Courtesy of Maggie's)

Figure 6.3 Planimetric diagramme of the Church of Fratte (1974) by Paolo Portoghesi, used by Rudolf Arnheim in his book (1977) to represent a phenomenal field generated by forces released by the curved walls (Courtesy of Paolo Portoghesi)

Figures 6.4 and 6.5 Maggie's West London (2008). Early floor plan sketch (Courtesy of RSHP). At Maggie's the idea of an interspersed continuity, a kind of evolving experience, is physically readable in obvious things like "the building as a grid" (©Marco Castelli Nirmal)

Figure 6.6 At Maggie's West London (2008), if we look up we can see a floating roof with lanterns framing the clouds visually mitigating the intrusive presence of the hospital (©Marco Castelli Nirmal)

Figure 6.7 At Maggie's the sequence of spaces divides or joins in a flexible way through sliding doors and movable walls 'which can be left a little open' (Maggie's West London, 2008) (©Marco Castelli Nirmal)

Figure 6.8 At Maggie's, stratifications of images are the essence of phenomenal transparency (Maggie's Glasgow, 2011) (©Marco Castelli Nirmal)

Figure 6.9 In a Maggie' centre, phenomenology is an indispensable condition for triggering psychological flexibility (Maggie's Oldham, 2017) (©Marco Castelli Nirmal)

Figure 7.1 Triangular diagramme of Maggie's Triad system showing a stable relational structure

Figure 7.2 Ground floor plan of Acute Mental Health Facility, City Hospital, Belfast (2019) designed by Richard Murphy Architects in association with RPP Architects (Drawings Courtesy of Richard Murphy Architects)

Appendices

11   Figure A_I1a, A_I1b, A_I1c, A_I1d, Architectural Brief (2007) (Courtesy of Maggie's)

12   Figure A_I2a, A_I2b, A_I2c, A_I2d, Architectural Brief (2007) (Courtesy of Maggie's)

13   Figure A_I3a, A_I3b, A_I3c, A_I3d, Architectural Brief (2007) (Courtesy of Maggie's)

14   Figure A_II Maggie's Support Programme (2007) (Courtesy of Maggie's)

15   Figure A_III 1, A_II 2 Maggie's Map and Timeline (1996 onwards) (Courtesy of Maggie's)

16   Figure A_IV The Maggie's centres Floorplans (1996 onwards) (Courtesy of Maggie's)

17   Figure A_V Users' Taxonomy of feelings (©author)

INDEX

Note: *Italic* page numbers refer to figures.